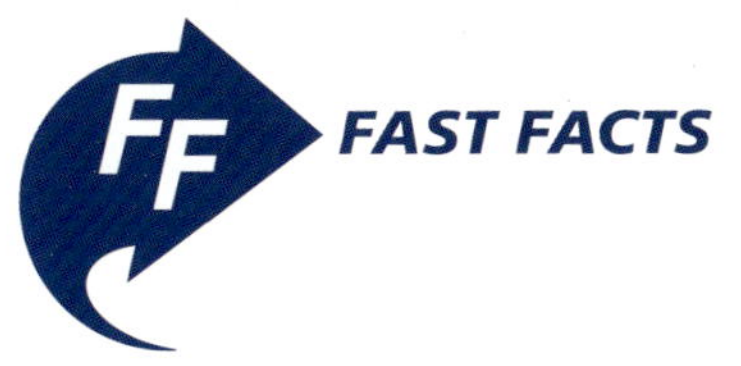

Thrombotic Thrombocytopenic Purpura

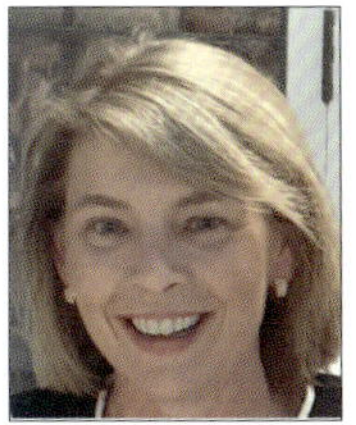

Marie A Scully MD
Department of Haematology
University College London Hospitals
NHS Foundation Trust
London, UK

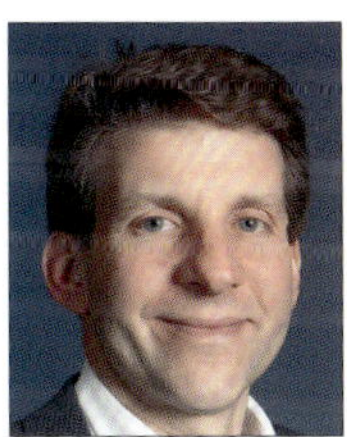

Spero R Cataland MD
Department of Hematology
Ohio State University, Columbus
Ohio, USA

Declaration of Independence
This book is as balanced and as practical as we can make it.
Ideas for improvement are always welcome: fastfacts@karger.com

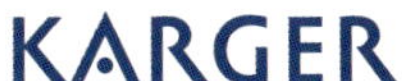

Fast Facts: Thrombotic Thrombocytopenic Purpura
First published 2020

S. Karger Publishers Limited, Elizabeth House, Queen Street,
Abingdon, Oxford OX14 3LN, UK
Tel: +44 (0)1235 523233

Book orders can be placed by telephone (+41 61 306 1440)
or email (orders@karger.com), or via the website at: karger.com
Fast Facts is a trademark of S. Karger Publishers Limited.

A CIP record for this title is available from the British Library.

ISBN 978-1-912776-79-5

Scully MA (Marie)
Fast Facts: Thrombotic Thrombocytopenic Purpura/Marie A Scully, Spero R Cataland

Medical illustrations by Graeme Chambers.
Typesetting by Thomas Bohm, User Design, Illustration and Typesetting, UK.

Printed in the UK with Xpedient Print.

Made possible by an unrestricted educational grant from Ablynx, a Sanofi company. Ablynx did not have any influence on the content and all items were subject to independent peer and editorial review.

List of abbreviations 4

Introduction 5

Disease overview 7

Clinical presentation 12

Differential diagnosis 25

Laboratory findings and diagnosis 38

Management 48

Useful resources 57

Index 59

Abbreviations

ADAMTS13: ADAM metallopeptidase with thrombospondin type 1 motif 13

aHUS: atypical hemolytic uremic syndrome

ANA: antinuclear antibody

APTT: activated partial thromboplastin time

CBC: complete blood count

CFH: complement factor H

cTTP: congenital thrombotic thrombocytopenic purpura

DAT: direct antiglobulin test

DIC: disseminated intravascular coagulation

HAART: highly active antiretroviral therapies

HELLP: hemolysis, elevated liver enzymes and low platelet count

HIT: heparin-induced thrombocytopenia

HLH: hemophagocytic lymphohistiocytosis

HUS: hemolytic uremic syndrome

IgG: immunoglobulin G

ITP: immune thrombocytopenia

iTTP: immune-mediated thrombotic thrombocytopenic purpura

LDH: lactate dehydrogenase

MAHA: microangiopathic hemolytic anemia

MCV: mean cell volume

PT: prothrombin time

SLE: systemic lupus erythematosus

STEC: Shiga toxin-producing *Escherichia coli*

TMA: thrombotic microangiopathy

TTP: thrombotic thrombocytopenic purpura

UL-VWF: ultra-large von Willebrand factor

VWF: von Willebrand factor

Introduction

Thrombotic thrombocytopenic purpura (TTP) is a rare disorder of the blood coagulation system. In most cases, a lack of the ADAMTS13 enzyme leads to an accumulation of ultra-large von Willebrand factor molecules in the plasma which, in turn, initiate the formation of microscopic thromboses in small blood vessels. TTP is a medical emergency. Timely diagnosis and urgent and effective management are vital – mortality in those untreated is in the region of 90%.

The understanding of TTP pathogenesis has increased markedly in recent decades. It is now known that TTP is acquired (immune-mediated) or congenital, and that the most common type – the acquired form – predominantly affects women in their 40s. It is also clear that the prompt delivery of plasma exchange saves lives.

Fast Facts: Thrombotic Thrombocytopenic Purpura sets out, in a clear and accessible format, the steps to suspecting, diagnosing and treating this potentially devastating disease. These steps are complemented by clear descriptions of the disease mechanism and epidemiology. Differential diagnosis, which is of the utmost importance for this disease, is explored in detail.

Whether you work in hematology, neurology, nephrology, gastroenterology or the emergency department, you may encounter a person with TTP. Our aim is to equip you with, or remind you of, the knowledge you need to recognize this disease and treat it swiftly.

1 Disease overview

Matthew Stubbs MD, University College London Hospitals NHS Foundation Trust, London, UK

Thrombotic thrombocytopenic purpura (TTP) is a life-threatening microangiopathy characterized by thrombocytopenia, microangiopathic hemolytic anemia (MAHA) and organ ischemia related to platelet-rich thrombi.[1] TTP exists as both an acquired, immune-mediated form and an inherited form.

In acquired TTP, there is an immune-mediated deficiency of ADAM metallopeptidase with thrombospondin type 1 motif 13 (ADAMTS13; a disintegrin and metalloprotease with thrombospondin type 1 repeats, Figure 1.1), with levels below 10 IU/dL.[1]

In congenital TTP (cTTP), an inherited deficiency in ADAMTS13 (usually to undetectable levels) is caused by homozygous or compound heterozygous mutations in the *ADAMTS13* gene (in a compound heterozygous mutation there are two different mutant alleles at a particular gene locus, one on each chromosome of the pair).[2–5] Congenital TTP is also known as Upshaw–Schulman syndrome or hereditary or familial TTP.

TTP should be differentiated from hemolytic uremic syndrome (HUS) and other thrombotic microangiopathies, as these disorders may have similar presenting features but, importantly, do not have ADAMTS13 deficiency.[1]

Epidemiology

It has been estimated that the incidence of immune-mediated TTP (iTTP) and cTTP is 2–6 per million, with cTTP accounting for 2–10% of cases in international registries.[6]

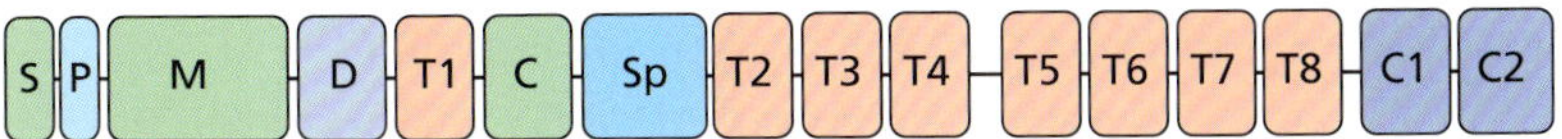

Figure 1.1 The ADAMTS13 protein, which is lacking in thrombotic thrombocytopenic purpura. C, cysteine rich; C1 and 2, CUB 1 and 2; D, disintegrin; M, metalloprotease; P, propeptide; S, signal peptide; Sp, spacer; T1–8, thrombospondin repeats 1–8.

Immune-mediated TTP. The reported annual incidence is 6 per million (UK TTP Registry) and 1.74 per million (Oklahoma TTP-HUS Registry). Individuals with iTTP tend to be young women; the median age is 43 years and there is a female predominance of 73%. The major ethnic groups affected by TTP in the UK are white (64%) and African-Caribbean (27%).[7,8] The etiology of most iTTP is primarily idiopathic (76%); secondary precipitants include infection, associated autoimmune disease, pregnancy, HIV and, rarely, drugs.[7,8]

Congenital TTP is also an ultra-rare disorder with, in the last 15 years, 73 confirmed cases described in the UK TTP Registry.[6] An additional 123 cases have been identified in the international Hereditary TTP Registry.[9] Individuals from Europe, Asia, the Americas and Africa have been enrolled in the international Hereditary TTP Registry, with first disease recognition recorded between birth and 70 years. The Registry has detected 98 different *ADAMTS13* mutations (see below).[9]

Etiology

Immune-mediated TTP results from an acquired deficiency of a cleaving protease for von Willebrand factor (VWF),[10,11] now identified as ADAMTS13.[4] This severe deficiency of ADAMTS13 function can result in the accumulation of ultra-large VWF (UL-VWF) in the plasma, which tethers platelets and results in platelet-rich thrombi within the endothelial surface of the microcirculation (Figure 1.2). These microthrombi can affect multiple organ systems, leading to tissue injury and a MAHA.

The mechanism of ADAMTS13 deficiency is autoimmune, with autoantibodies (typically immunoglobulin [Ig]G) targeting ADAMTS13. Antibodies can target different domains of ADAMTS13, but most people have antibodies that bind epitopes in the N-terminal domain.[12–16] The main mechanism by which autoantibodies contribute to ADAMTS13 deficiency is thought to be direct inhibition of ADAMTS13, but increased clearance of ADAMTS13 also contributes.

Congenital TTP. In contrast to iTTP, the mechanism of ADAMTS13 deficiency in cTTP is through mutations within the *ADAMTS13* gene itself. *ADAMTS13* is located on chromosome 9q34, containing

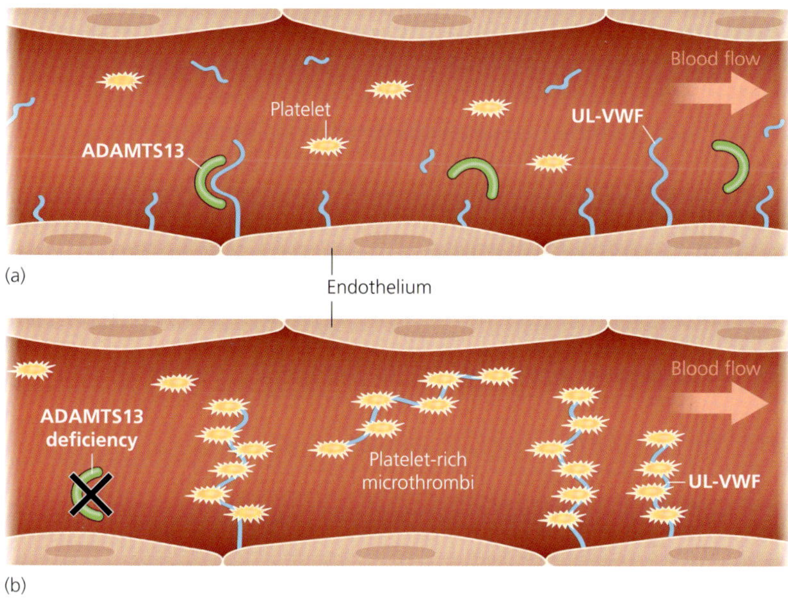

Figure 1.2 (a) Normal cleavage of ultra-large von Willebrand factor (UL-VWF) in the presence of ADAMTS13. (b) Platelet-rich microthrombi form if ADAMTS13 is deficient.

29 exons and encompassing 1427 amino acids.[6,9,17] The mutations are autosomal recessive, with individuals being either homozygous for a mutation (36%) or a compound heterozygote (64%); the main disease-causing mutations are frameshift, missense and nonsense. Mutations have been reported throughout the *ADAMTS13* gene.[6,9,17] Importantly, in cTTP there is no functional inhibitor of the ADAMTS13 protease.

There are typically two peaks seen in clinical presentation: one in childhood, with a median age of 3.5 years; and one in adulthood, which is typically related to pregnancy (median age 31 years) – in individuals who present in adulthood, 69% of cases are associated with pregnancy.[6] The type of mutation identified has been shown to differ between age groups, with pre-spacer domain mutations (see Figure 1.1) leading to earlier symptom development in childhood.[6]

The most commonly reported mutation in the UK is rs142572218 (exon 24 R1060W missense mutation), which typically has a later onset of presentation.[6] The international Hereditary TTP Registry found the most common mutation to be rs387906343 (exon 29, c.4143_4144dupA, p.Glu1382Argfs*6). A larger proportion of compound heterozygous carriers of c.4143_4144dupA (p.Glu1382ArgfsTer6) have overt disease before 3 months of age compared with carriers of homozygous mutations.[9]

Key points – disease overview

- Thrombotic thrombocytopenic purpura (TTP) exists as immune-mediated (autoimmune) and congenital forms.
- TTP is mediated by a deficiency of ADAMTS13.
- ADAMTS13 deficiency leads to accumulation of ultra-large von Willebrand factor, causing multisystem microthrombi.
- Congenital TTP has two incidence peaks, first in childhood and then in adulthood, typically in pregnancy.

References

1. Scully M, Cataland S, Coppo P et al. Consensus on the standardization of terminology in thrombotic thrombocytopenic purpura and related thrombotic microangiopathies. *J Thromb Haemost* 2017;15:312–22.

2. Camilleri RS, Scully M, Thomas M et al. A phenotype-genotype correlation of ADAMTS13 mutations in congenital thrombotic thrombocytopenic purpura patients treated in the United Kingdom. *J Thromb Haemost* 2012;10: 1792–1801.

3. Lotta LA, Garagiola I, Palla R et al. ADAMTS13 mutations and polymorphisms in congenital thrombotic thrombocytopenic purpura. *Hum Mutat* 2010;31:11–19.

4. Levy GG, Nichols WC, Lian EC et al. Mutations in a member of the ADAMTS gene family cause thrombotic thrombocytopenic purpura. *Nature* 2001;413:488–94.

5. Schneppenheim R, Budde U, Oyen F et al. Von Willebrand factor cleaving protease and ADAMTS13 mutations in childhood TTP. *Blood* 2003;101:1845–50.

6. Alwan F, Vendramin C, Liesner R et al. Characterization and treatment of congenital thrombotic thrombocytopenic purpura. *Blood* 2019;133:1644–51.

7. Scully M, Yarranton H, Liesner R et al. Regional UK TTP Registry: correlation with laboratory ADAMTS 13 analysis and clinical features. *Br J Haematol* 2008;142:819–26.

8. Coppo P, Schwarzinger M, Buffet M et al. Predictive features of severe acquired ADAMTS13 deficiency in idiopathic thrombotic microangiopathies: the French TMA reference center experience. *PLoS One* 2010;5:e10208.

9. van Dorland HA, Taleghani MM, Sakai K et al. The international Hereditary Thrombotic Thrombocytopenic Purpura Registry: key findings at enrolment until 2017. *Haematologica* 2019;104:2107–15.

10. Furlan M, Robles R, Galbusera M et al. Von Willebrand factor-cleaving protease in thrombotic thrombocytopenic purpura and the hemolytic-uremic syndrome. *N Engl J Med* 1998;339:1578–84.

11. Tsai HM, Lian ECY. Antibodies to von Willebrand factor-cleaving protease in acute thrombotic thrombocytopenic purpura. *N Engl J Med* 1998;339:1585–94.

12. Thomas MR, de Groot R, Scully MA et al. Pathogenicity of anti-ADAMTS13 autoantibodies in acquired thrombotic thrombocytopenic purpura. *EBioMedicine* 2015;2:942–52.

13. Joly BS, Coppo P, Veyradier A. Thrombotic thrombocytopenic purpura. *Blood* 2017;129:2836–46.

14. Pos W, Crawley JTB, Fijnheer R et al. An autoantibody epitope comprising residues R660, Y661, and Y665 in the ADAMTS13 spacer domain identifies a binding site for the A2 domain of VWF. *Blood* 2010;115:1640–9.

15. Zheng XL, Wu HM, Shang D et al. Multiple domains of ADAMTS13 are targeted by autoantibodies against ADAMTS13 in patients with acquired idiopathic thrombotic thrombocytopenic purpura. *Haematologica* 2010;95:1555–62.

16. Pos W, Sorvillo N, Fijnheer R et al. Residues arg568 and phe592 contribute to an antigenic surface for anti-ADAMTS13 antibodies in the spacer domain. *Haematologica* 2011;96:1670–7.

17. Fujimura Y, Matsumoto M, Isonishi A et al. Natural history of Upshaw-Schulman syndrome based on ADAMTS13 gene analysis in Japan. *J Thromb Haemost* 2011;9(Suppl 1):283–301.

2 Clinical presentation

Lucy Naeve MD, University College London Hospitals
NHS Foundation Trust, London, UK

Historically, thrombotic thrombocytopenic purpura (TTP) was characterized by the 'pentad' of fever, microangiopathic hemolytic anemia (MAHA), thrombocytopenia, neurological symptoms and renal impairment.[1] It is now well recognized that only a small minority (in the region of 5%)[2] of episodes feature all aspects of the pentad simultaneously and that clinical presentations are diverse.

Classic presentation of acute TTP

Various international and national TTP registries have allowed us to understand how TTP typically presents. The most common presentation of acute TTP is a previously healthy young to middle-aged adult with MAHA, severe thrombocytopenia and features of end-organ damage. There is a consensus that overall women are roughly twice as commonly affected by TTP as men, though Japanese data are unusual in showing a 1:1 ratio.[3]

There are a large variety of possible presenting symptoms, which can be categorized into those resulting from: (1) MAHA; (2) thrombocytopenia; (3) end-organ microvascular thrombosis; and (4) other (Figure 2.1). The frequencies of various symptoms at presentation according to data from six of the larger and more recently published registries are summarized in Table 2.1.[2–8] The end organs most commonly affected are the brain, heart, kidneys and gastrointestinal tract.

Non-specific symptoms such as malaise, fatigue and weakness are common, and a non-specific prodrome may often precede the onset of the more specific features of hemolysis, thrombocytopenia or end-organ damage. In terms of end-organ manifestations, neurological symptoms appear to be the most predominant according to the published data, though these can be as subtle as headache and mild cognitive impairment. While the heart is probably the next most commonly involved organ, with an elevated cardiac troponin in approximately 60% of individuals,[9,10] this is usually subclinical and only a minority (10–14%)[5,10] present with cardiac symptoms.

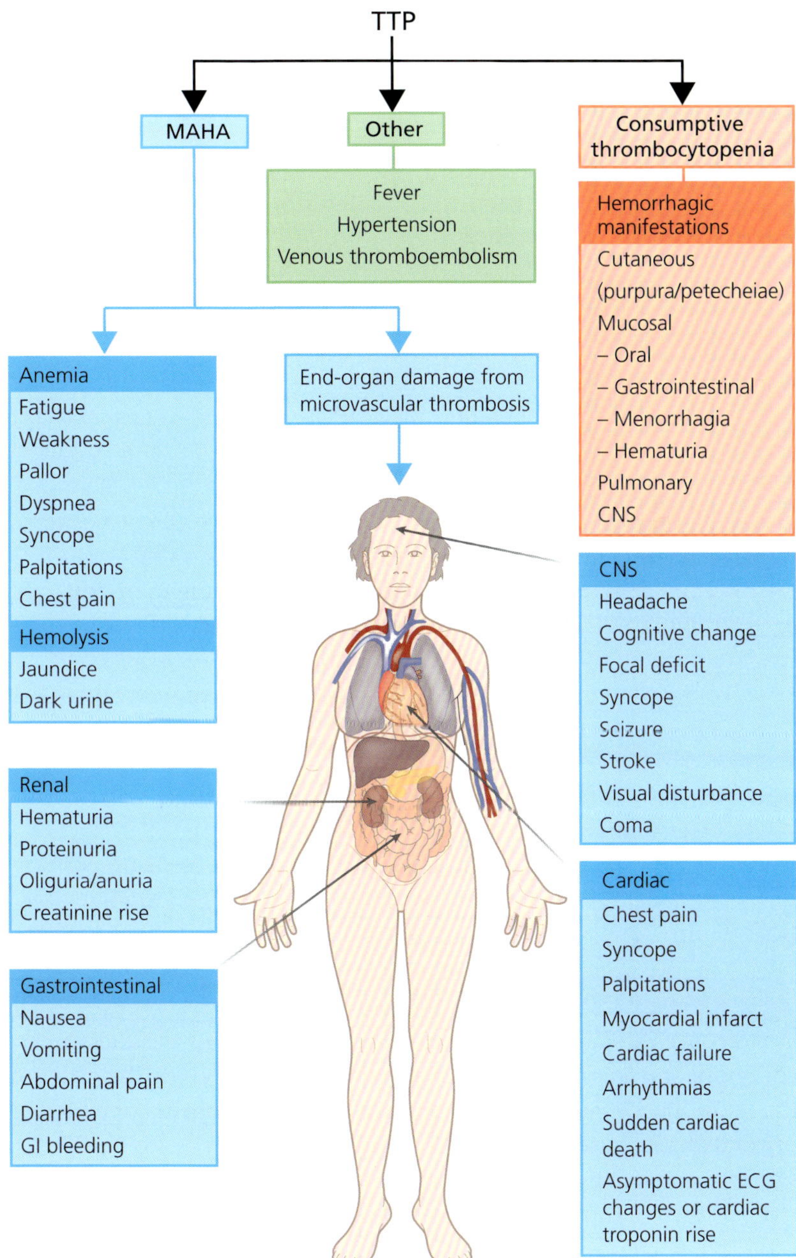

Figure 2.1 Potential presenting symptoms of TTP. CNS, central nervous system; ECG, electrocardiogram; GI, gastrointestinal; MAHA, microangiopathic hemolytic anemia.

TABLE 2.1

Frequencies of various presenting features of acute TTP according to international registries

Characteristic	TMA Registry of French Reference Center[4]	Milan TTP Registry[5]	Regional UK TTP Registry[6]
Number of patients included	772	302	176 (236*)
Cohort	Adult-onset, acquired and congenital (3%)	Adult- and childhood-onset, acquired only	Adult- and childhood-onset, acquired and congenital (5%)
Bleeding (%)	N/A	68	~ 60
Neurological (%)	61 (30% headache or confusion; 31% coma, seizures, stroke, TIA)	43	78 (10% coma)
GI (%)	35	N/A	35
Cardiac (%)	N/A	10	42 (including asymptomatic troponin rise/ ECG changes)
Renal (%)	40% renal insufficiency; 10% acute renal failure	18 (4% with creatinine ≥ 221 μmol/L‡)	1/3 had elevated creatinine
Fever (%)	40	N/A	21
Other			

*Number of acute episodes. †1.5 mg/dL. ‡2.5 mg/dL.

ECG, electrocardiogram; GI, gastrointestinal; N/A, data not available; TIA, transient ischemic attack; TMA, thrombotic microangiopathy; VTE, venous thromboembolism.

Japanese cohort[3]	Oklahoma TTP Registry[2,7]	Australian TTP/TMA Registry[8]
186	78,[7] 65[2]	57 (72*)
Adult- and childhood-onset, acquired idiopathic only	Adult- and childhood-onset, acquired only	Adult- and childhood-onset, acquired and congenital
N/A	54[2]	46
79	52 (32% 'major' [coma, seizure, stroke, focal symptoms]; 20% minor [e.g. confusion, headache])[7]	71 (42% headache, 28% cognitive change, 24% focal deficit, 8% seizure, 6% stroke)
N/A	69[2]	39
N/A	N/A	3 ('thrombotic')
76 (elevated creatinine or abnormal urinalysis)	47 with creatinine ≥ 132.6 μmol/L[†] (14% ≥ 221 μmol/L[‡])	10 (including hematuria, oligo/anuria, fluid overload and 'other')
72	N/A	28
	Weakness/fatigue in 63%	VTE 6%

Renal symptoms. The frequency of renal manifestations cited in the literature varies considerably, most likely because of the different definitions of renal involvement. However, there is a consensus that renal impairment, if present, is usually mild, and that acute renal failure requiring renal replacement therapy normally favors a diagnosis of atypical (or Shiga toxin-associated) hemolytic uremic syndrome (HUS) over TTP. Testing for ADAMTS13 should be performed regardless, as there are reports of end-stage renal failure in TTP, particularly in congenital TTP (cTTP).[11,12]

Gastrointestinal symptoms, presumably resulting from intestinal ischemia, are also commonly reported in TTP. The presence of diarrhea – even bloody, though this is classically associated with Shiga toxin-associated HUS – should not delay ADAMTS13 testing.

Other symptoms. In addition to the specific manifestations of TTP, individuals may demonstrate features of an underlying cause or trigger (though more than 50% of cases are idiopathic[13]). Examples include features of infection (12.7–27%);[4,5,8] autoimmune disease (especially systemic lupus erythematosus [SLE], see page 30); HIV infection; pregnancy or hormonal medication; and recent initiation of a causative drug.

Atypical presentations in adulthood

The spectrum of severity of presentation in TTP is marked. Some individuals can appear remarkably 'well' or even asymptomatic[14] when MAHA and thrombocytopenia are first detected. Equally important to bear in mind is that clinical deterioration can be alarmingly rapid, and it can include sudden unexpected cardiac arrest.[14]

Although TTP usually first presents in young to middle-aged adults, de novo presentation in the elderly is seen. Japanese data reveal first presentation of immune-mediated TTP (iTTP) in individuals up to 87 years old, with evidence of higher short-term mortality in those presenting at older ages.[3]

Childhood and adolescent onset

Onset of TTP in childhood or adolescence is also seen, though less commonly than in adulthood, accounting for approximately 10% of all first presentations of TTP.[13] The major difference is the higher proportion of cTTP cases. While about 98% of cases of TTP presenting in adulthood are immune-mediated, only about two-thirds of cases of childhood-onset TTP are immune-mediated.[13]

The presentation of cTTP is discussed on pages 18–20. The presentation of iTTP in children and adolescents was the subject of a French series of 45 cases.[15] Girls were 2.5 times more commonly affected than boys, with an overall median age at onset of 13 years (range 4 months–17 years). In 56% of cases there was an underlying cause, such as infection (18%) or autoimmunity (17%). The clinical presentation mirrored that seen in adults, with MAHA and thrombocytopenia (usually severe) in all cases, fever in 36% and end-organ ischemic damage in 64%. The pattern of affected organs differed slightly from that in adults: renal insult was most common (42%), followed by brain (40%) and with cardiac injury in only 7%.

Association with other autoimmune diseases

Given the tendency for autoimmune diseases to cluster in affected individuals, it is perhaps unsurprising that people with iTTP have been shown to be at increased risk of other autoimmune conditions. A cross-sectional study of the TMA Registry of the French Reference Center revealed other autoimmune diagnoses in 22% of 261 patients,[16] similar to the 20% recorded in 302 Milan TTP Registry cases.[5] In the French data, 43% of other autoimmune diagnoses predated the diagnosis of TTP, while 28% were diagnosed simultaneously, and 28% after TTP (up to 12 years after).

The most commonly associated autoimmune condition is SLE. The French study revealed 26 cases of SLE in 261 cases of TTP.[16] In addition, 58% of TTP cases were positive for antinuclear antibodies (ANA) (> 1:80) at the time of TTP diagnosis, though the presence of double-stranded (ds)DNA was more strongly associated with the development of another autoimmune disorder following the diagnosis of TTP.

Associations with Sjögren's syndrome,[16] rheumatoid arthritis and systemic sclerosis,[17] antiphospholipid syndrome[4] and Hashimoto's thyroiditis, immune thrombocytopenia (ITP), psoriasis and celiac disease[18] have also been reported.

Not all cases of thrombotic microangiopathy associated with connective tissue disorders are TTP, however: in a Japanese series of 127 cases, only a minority had severe ADAMTS13 deficiency.[19]

Congenital (hereditary) TTP

In contrast to the typical onset in adulthood of iTTP, the rarer congenital form of TTP (accounting for about 5% of all cases of TTP), has classically been associated with an acute onset in the neonatal period or childhood. However, through the analysis of registry data,[12,20,21] it is now well established that clinical presentation is diverse, with a substantial proportion of cTTP cases actually presenting in adulthood, especially in the context of pregnancy.

While all cases have persistent severe deficiency of ADAMTS13, additional triggers such as infection or pregnancy are required to provoke acute symptoms of overt TTP. Rarer triggers include alcohol excess, medication, illicit drug use or injury. Broadly speaking, the acute phase is characterized by MAHA, thrombocytopenia and end-organ damage in a similar fashion to iTTP. The frequency of acute episodes varies considerably between individuals, depending on exposure to triggers, treatment and underlying (poorly understood) disease factors. Some may develop frequent relapses, often without clear triggers, while others may develop a state of persistent disease activity with MAHA, thrombocytopenia and progressive end-organ damage.[22]

Childhood- versus adult-onset of cTTP. Of 73 UK TTP Registry cases of cTTP, 38% initially presented in childhood/adolescence,[8] as did 58% of 43 Japanese cases.[21] Presentations in this period range from neonatal jaundice due to Coombs-negative hemolysis (often requiring exchange transfusion) and thrombocytopenia (seen in 42% of 43 Japanese cases[21]) to later presentations with thrombocytopenia with varying degrees of MAHA, often triggered by infection.[20]

Meanwhile, 62% of cases of cTTP in the UK Registry were diagnosed in adulthood, with a median age at diagnosis of 31 years.[20] Of note, just over two-thirds of these diagnoses in adulthood were associated with pregnancy. In adulthood, cTTP usually presents with overt thrombotic microangiopathy, though the diagnosis is sometimes made as a result of investigations for thrombocytopenia.

There is a distinction to be made between 'true' adult-onset cTTP, where the first episode of overt TTP occurs in adulthood (often triggered by pregnancy) and late recognition of cTTP during adulthood. In the latter scenario of delayed diagnosis, previous incorrect diagnoses such as chronic ITP or Evans syndrome may have been made. There may also be a history of stroke or pregnancy losses, or evidence of chronic end-organ damage including cardiac and renal dysfunction, especially if the diagnosis is made in late adulthood. Diagnosis in late adulthood does not always imply delayed diagnosis, however: two male patients in the Japanese series developed sudden overt TTP aged 55 and 63 years with no apparent abnormalities on preceding annual health examinations.[21]

International and national registry data illustrate the lack of a clear correlation between residual ADAMTS13 activity and timing of onset: of those with ADAMTS13 activity below 1 IU/dL, 40% had a neonatal onset of disease but 20% seemed to present at ages over 20 years.[12] Genotype–phenotype associations may be of relevance. For example, compound heterozygote carriers of *ADAMTS13* c.4143_4144dupA mutations, observed most frequently in the international Hereditary TTP Registry, tended to have an earlier presentation than those with a homozygous mutation.

End-organ damage in cTTP

The pattern of ischemic end-organ involvement mirrors that of iTTP, in terms of mainly affecting the brain, heart and kidneys. Arterial thrombotic events occur in all age groups, and more than 50% of those aged over 40 years in the international Hereditary TTP Registry had experienced at least one episode.[12] Stroke or transient ischemic attack was a complication in 31% of the cases included in the international Registry and 27% of UK TTP Registry patients.[20] Neurocognitive sequelae such as depression and memory impairment are also reported. Myocardial infarction is less commonly seen than cerebrovascular involvement. International registry data also suggest that chronic renal impairment may be more prominent than in iTTP, with 25% having renal insufficiency at the time of enrolment and 12.5% having required renal replacement therapy.

Subacute features of cTTP

A key difference between cTTP and iTTP is that untreated cTTP is frequently associated with insidious but often debilitating chronic symptoms such as headaches, lethargy and abdominal pain, even in the absence of overt thrombocytopenia and MAHA.[20] These 'subacute' features often respond to plasma therapy, implying that they result from subclinical thrombotic microangiopathy (TMA) activity.

Presentation in pregnancy

Pregnancy is a well-established trigger for TTP, accounting for 5–10% of all cases of TTP in UK[6] and French[4] registries. Both immune and congenital forms are seen, but especially the latter. In all pregnancies, rising levels of von Willebrand factor (VWF) contribute to a fall in ADAMTS13 over the course of pregnancy and into the postpartum period.[23,24] In cases of TTP, however, ADAMTS13 activity falls to a critically low level. This can result in a first overt presentation of MAHA and thrombocytopenia in previously asymptomatic women with cTTP ('late-onset' cTTP), while women with a prior diagnosis of cTTP will usually experience an acute episode in pregnancy in the absence of prophylactic treatment. Meanwhile, pregnancy-induced changes may trigger iTTP.

Onset of TTP can occur throughout pregnancy and into the postpartum period. Presentation was commonest in the second trimester in 42 de novo presentations reported in the French registry,[25] whereas it was most common in the third trimester and postpartum period in 52 UK cases of de novo and relapsing TTP.[26] Of 42 French cases reported, 32 occurred in first pregnancies and 29 of the 42 had no discernible trigger other than pregnancy.

Presenting features are generally similar to those seen in non-pregnancy cases, though associated hypertension and proteinuria is often found,[26] which can lead, erroneously, to a diagnosis of pre-eclampsia.

Late-onset cTTP accounted for 66% (23/35) of UK cases of pregnancy-associated initial presentations of TTP and 24% (10/42) of French cases. Both figures are much higher than the proportion of cTTP in adult-onset TTP in general (approximately 5%). As is the case in non-pregnancy presentations, congenital cases cannot be distinguished from immune cases on the basis of clinical features alone. However, certain features may be more suggestive of a congenital etiology. First, cTTP nearly always presents in the first pregnancy, whereas iTTP can present initially in subsequent pregnancies. Second, in congenital cases, overt TMA may be preceded by isolated thrombocytopenia in the second to third trimesters.[21] Third, a predominance of neurological symptoms was described in UK congenital cases compared with immune-mediated cases.[26]

Fetal outcomes are unfortunately poor in the index pregnancies because of impairment of the uteroplacental circulation by platelet thrombi and ischemia, which can lead to severe fetal growth restriction and fetal loss. Live birth rates range between 31% and 58%,[25–27] with the worst outcomes seen for women presenting in the second trimester. However, prophylactic treatment in known cases of cTTP and close monitoring in women who have previously had an episode of iTTP can vastly improve fetal outcomes.[26]

Differential diagnosis. Given the above, TTP (especially previously undiagnosed congenital disease) should be considered in the differential diagnosis of unexplained fetal growth restriction, unexplained second trimester pregnancy losses, unexplained thrombocytopenia in pregnancy (beyond the level expected for gestational thrombocytopenia, for example below 75×10^9/L), 'atypical'/'severe' presentations of pre-eclampsia and in cases of HELLP syndrome (hemolysis, elevated liver enzymes and low platelet count), with a low threshold for ADAMTS13 activity testing in all of these scenarios.

Key points – clinical presentation

- Thrombotic thrombocytopenic purpura (TTP) usually presents acutely in previously healthy adults with diverse features resulting from microvascular thrombosis: (1) microangiopathic hemolytic anemia; (2) thrombocytopenia; and (3) end-organ damage.
- The brain, heart, kidneys and gastrointestinal tract are the most commonly affected end organs. Neurological symptoms are the most common.
- Congenital TTP is a much more common cause of TTP in childhood/adolescence and in pregnancy than in non-pregnant adults.
- Acute presentations of congenital TTP cannot generally be distinguished from immune-mediated TTP on the basis of presenting features, though some individuals have chronic subacute symptoms.
- Pregnancy is a trigger for TTP, especially the congenital form. This should be considered as a potential cause for unexplained fetal growth restriction or stillbirth, unexplained thrombocytopenia in pregnancy and atypical/severe cases of pre-eclampsia/HELLP syndrome (hemolysis, elevated liver enzymes and low platelet count).

References

1. Amorosi EL, Ultmann JE. Thrombotic thrombocytopenic purpura: report of 16 cases and review of the literature. *Medicine* 1966;45:139–60.

2. George JN. How I treat patients with thrombotic thrombocytopenic purpura: 2010. *Blood* 2010;116: 4060–9.

3. Matsumoto M, Bennett CL, Isonishi A et al. Acquired idiopathic ADAMTS13 activity deficient thrombotic thrombocytopenic purpura in a population from Japan. *PLoS One* 2012;7:e33029.

4. Mariotte E, Azoulay E, Galicier L et al. Epidemiology and pathophysiology of adulthood-onset thrombotic microangiopathy with severe ADAMTS13 deficiency (thrombotic thrombocytopenic purpura): a cross-sectional analysis of the French national registry for thrombotic microangiopathy. *Lancet Haematol* 2016;3:e237–45.

5. Mancini I, Pontiggia S, Palla R et al. Clinical and laboratory features of patients with acquired thrombotic thrombocytopenic purpura: fourteen years of the Milan TTP Registry. *Thromb Haemost* 2019;119:695–704.

6. Scully M, Yarranton H, Liesner R et al. Regional UK TTP registry: correlation with laboratory ADAMTS 13 analysis and clinical features. *Br J Haematol* 2008;142:819–26.

7. Page EE, Kremer Hovinga JA, Terrell DR et al. Thrombotic thrombocytopenic purpura: diagnostic criteria, clinical features, and long-term outcomes from 1995 through 2015. *Blood Adv* 2017;1: 590–600.

8. Blombery P, Kivivali L, Pepperell D et al. Diagnosis and management of thrombotic thrombocytopenic purpura (TTP) in Australia: findings from the first 5 years of the Australian TTP/thrombotic microangiopathy registry. *Int Med J* 2016;46:71–9.

9. Hughes C, McEwan JR, Longair I et al. Cardiac involvement in acute thrombotic thrombocytopenic purpura: association with troponin T and IgG antibodies to ADAMTS 13. *J Thromb Haemost* 2009;7:529–36.

10. Benhamou Y, Boelle PY, Baudin B et al. Cardiac troponin-I on diagnosis predicts early death and refractoriness in acquired thrombotic thrombocytopenic purpura. Experience of the French Thrombotic Microangiopathies Reference Center. *J Thromb Haemost* 2015;13:293–302.

11. Loirat C, Veyradier A, Girma JP et al. Thrombotic thrombocytopenic purpura associated with von Willebrand factor-cleaving protease (ADAMTS13) deficiency in children. *Semin Thromb Hemost* 2006;32:90–7.

12. van Dorland HA, Taleghani MM, Sakai K et al. The international Hereditary Thrombotic Thrombocytopenic Purpura Registry: key findings at enrollment until 2017. *Haematologica* 2019;104:2107–15.

13. Joly BS, Coppo P, Veyradier A. Thrombotic thrombocytopenic purpura. *Blood* 2017;129:2836–46.

14. George JN. The remarkable diversity of thrombotic thrombocytopenic purpura: a perspective. *Blood Adv* 2018;2: 1510–16.

15. Joly BS, Stepanian A, Leblanc T et al. Child-onset and adolescent-onset acquired thrombotic thrombocytopenic purpura with severe ADAMTS13 deficiency: a cohort study of the French national registry for thrombotic microangiopathy. *Lancet Haematol* 2016;3:e537–46.

16. Roriz M, Landais M, Desprez J et al. Risk factors for autoimmune diseases development after thrombotic thrombocytopenic purpura. *Medicine* 2015;94:e1598.

17. Kremer Hovinga JA, Coppo P, Lammle B et al. Thrombotic thrombocytopenic purpura. *Nat Rev Dis Primers* 2017;3:17020.

18. John ML, Scharrer I. Autoimmune disorders in patients with idiopathic thrombotic thrombocytopenic purpura. *Hamostaseologie* 2012;32(Suppl 1):S86–9.

19. Matsuyama T, Kuwana M, Matsumoto M et al. Heterogeneous pathogenic processes of thrombotic microangiopathies in patients with connective tissue diseases. *Thromb Haemost* 2009;102:371–8.

20. Alwan F, Vendramin C, Liesner R et al. Characterization and treatment of congenital thrombotic thrombocytopenic purpura. *Blood* 2019;133:1644–51.

21. Fujimura Y, Matsumoto M, Isonishi A et al. Natural history of Upshaw-Schulman syndrome based on ADAMTS13 gene analysis in Japan. *J Thromb Haemost* 2011;9(Suppl 1):283–301.

22. Krogh AS, Waage A, Quist-Paulsen P. Congenital thrombotic thrombocytopenic purpura. *Tidsskr Nor Laegeforen* 2016;136:1452–7.

23. Mannucci PM, Canciani MT, Forza I et al. Changes in health and disease of the metalloprotease that cleaves von Willebrand factor. *Blood* 2001;98:2730–5.

24. Sanchez-Luceros A, Farias CE, Amaral MM et al. von Willebrand factor-cleaving protease (ADAMTS13) activity in normal non-pregnant women, pregnant and post-delivery women. *Thromb Haemost* 2004;92:1320–6.

25. Moatti-Cohen M, Garrec C, Wolf M et al. Unexpected frequency of Upshaw-Schulman syndrome in pregnancy-onset thrombotic thrombocytopenic purpura. *Blood* 2012;119:5888–97.

26. Scully M, Thomas M, Underwood M et al. Thrombotic thrombocytopenic purpura and pregnancy: presentation, management, and subsequent pregnancy outcomes. *Blood* 2014;124:211–19.

27. Fujimura Y, Matsumoto M, Kokame K et al. Pregnancy-induced thrombocytopenia and TTP, and the risk of fetal death, in Upshaw-Schulman syndrome: a series of 15 pregnancies in 9 genotyped patients. *Br J Haematol* 2009;144:742–54.

3 Differential diagnosis

Karim Attia MD, OhioHealth Hospitalist Medicine Service, Columbus, OH, USA

It is important to develop a broad differential when considering a potential diagnosis of thrombotic thrombocytopenic purpura (TTP) given the differing conditions that may present with thrombotic microangiopathy (TMA) findings (Table 3.1). The approach to differential diagnosis is summarized in Figure 3.1, at the end of this chapter.

TMA is a specific pathology within the microvasculature that leads to microvascular thrombosis which, in turn, causes a microangiopathic hemolytic anemia (MAHA), thrombocytopenia and, potentially, organ damage. The category of TMA includes the diagnoses of TTP, hemolytic uremic syndrome (HUS) and secondary thrombotic microangiopathies. TTP itself can be subdivided into immune-mediated TTP (iTTP) and congenital TTP (cTTP) (Upshaw–Schulman syndrome) – see chapter 1. HUS is divided into Shiga toxin-producing *Escherichia coli*-HUS (STEC-HUS, also referred to as typical or diarrhea-associated HUS) and atypical or complement-mediated HUS (aHUS).

Immune-mediated TTP

The hallmark of iTTP is the finding of thrombocytopenia and MAHA (including schistocytes and polychromasia) in the peripheral blood without an alternative clinical explanation. Although mild or moderate renal insufficiency can be seen in iTTP patients, the development of acute renal failure is rare and is more likely with other TMAs, particularly HUS. Clinical overlap can occur between these conditions and definitive laboratory testing can be time-consuming at a time when patients are usually critically ill and require immediate treatment. Therefore, in many cases, empiric treatment with plasma exchange prior to definitive diagnosis is the standard of care.

STEC-HUS (typical or diarrhea-associated HUS)

HUS is defined by the simultaneous occurrence of TMA with acute kidney injury. Renal involvement is typically much more severe than

TABLE 3.1

Differential diagnosis for individuals presenting with a thrombotic microangiopathy

Undetectable ADAMTS13 activity

- Immune-mediated TTP
- Congenital TTP

ADAMTS13 activity ≥ 20 IU/dL

- STEC-HUS
- aHUS
- Secondary TMA
  - Drug-induced
  - Disseminated intravascular coagulation
  - Systemic infection
  - Post-transplant
  - Cancer
  - Pregnancy-associated TMA
  - Autoimmune disorders
  - Cobalamin metabolic defects

aHUS, atypical hemolytic uremic syndrome; STEC-HUS, Shiga toxin-producing *Escherichia coli*-hemolytic uremic syndrome; TMA, thrombotic microangiopathy.

with TTP and the patient often presents with oliguria or anuria.[1] Traditionally, HUS was divided into diarrhea-positive and diarrhea-negative, but this is now known to be inaccurate as patients with aHUS may also present with diarrhea. A more accurate classification came about after better understanding of the pathophysiology that underpins a division into HUS (endothelial injury mediated by Shiga toxin) and secondary HUS or TMAs. Causes of secondary TMAs include severe infection with *Streptococcus pneumoniae*, HIV infection, drug toxicity (especially in people with cancer or following solid-organ transplant) and, rarely, autoimmune disorders such as systemic lupus erythematosus (SLE).

STEC-HUS is the most common form of HUS. It is primarily caused by STEC infection (*E. coli* O157:H7) and less frequently by infection with *Shigella dysenteriae* type 1 or other *E. coli* subtypes. It can occur at any age, but it usually affects children younger than 5 years. It can occur sporadically or as an epidemic and is associated with ingestion of contaminated food or water. STEC colonizes the gut, damages the epithelium and secretes Shiga toxin (Stx), which gets delivered to target organs. The tendency to cause renal failure lies in the fact that renal cells have a surface rich in globotriaosylceramide (Gb3), which binds the pentameric B subunit of Stx. Stx is then endocytosed, its A subunit is released and apoptotic cell death occurs. Patients usually develop abdominal pain, diarrhea (often bloody), followed by an acute TMA and renal injury within 5–13 days after the onset of diarrhea.[1] The TMA most commonly follows recovery from the acute diarrheal illness. ADAMTS13 levels should be normal in these cases.[2] STEC can be recovered by culturing stool on selective media[1] or it can be diagnosed through serologic testing. Treatment is usually supportive and includes intravenous fluids and transfusion support. Antibiotics early in the course of the STEC infection may actually increase the risk of HUS development.[3] Antimotility agents and nephrotoxic drugs should be avoided.

Atypical HUS

Atypical HUS refers to an acute TMA mediated by dysregulation of the complement system, typically the alternative pathway of complement activation (i.e. this is TMA that is not due to a secondary cause such as Stx).[4] Etiologies for aHUS include complement gene mutations (complement factor H [CFH] has the most common and most severe mutation) and antibodies to CFH that lead to an inability to control complement activation after it has been triggered for a normal physiological reason (for example, infection, pregnancy). Mutations may also affect complement factor I, membrane cofactor protein (CD46), C3 or factor B. Rarer causes of acute TMAs in children include mutation of *DGKE*, which encodes diacylglycerol kinase ε, and inborn errors of cobalamin C metabolism.

Atypical HUS is rare, with an incidence of 2 per million adults and 3.3 per million children under the age of 10.[5] Presentation can be similar to that of STEC-HUS, with acute renal failure and acute TMA findings. Classically, the presence of neurological symptoms was thought to be in favor of a diagnosis of TTP and profound renal failure in favor of aHUS. However, this has been shown to be unreliable in differentiating between the two, as patients with aHUS may present with neurological injury.[6] One reliable marker to differentiate aHUS from TTP is ADAMTS13 activity, which should be normal (non-deficient, typically > 20 IU/dL) in aHUS and undetectable (< 10 IU/dL) in TTP. A definitive diagnosis of aHUS can be confirmed by detection of complement gene mutations or antibodies to factor H if present, but up to 40% of individuals with aHUS may not have a detectable complement mutation.

Patients may be treated empirically with plasma exchange while awaiting the results of pretreatment ADAMTS13 activity to exclude a diagnosis of TTP. One-third of patients will respond completely to plasma exchange therapy, both hematologically and with end-organ response. If the response to plasma exchange is poor or partial (improvement in hemolytic parameters but no improvement in renal injury) after 4–5 days, plasma exchange should be stopped and eculizumab treatment should be initiated for a presumed diagnosis of aHUS.[6] Eculizumab works by binding to the terminal complement protein C5 and in so doing prevents the formation of the membrane attack complex, which is a barrier to further tissue injury.[7]

Drug-induced TMA

Many drugs have been associated with TMA findings, but use of quinine, ciclosporin and tacrolimus underlies 60% of cases.[8]

Quinine works via an immune mechanism that induces severe TMA, mainly in women, and it occurs suddenly – within a few hours of ingestion – causing constitutional symptoms, rash and oliguric renal failure. Injury occurs via quinine-dependent antibodies against platelets, endothelial and other cell types. ADAMTS13 levels are typically normal.[9] Most patients recover normal renal function within several weeks simply by stopping the drug and with supportive care.

Ciclosporin and tacrolimus can lead to the development of TMA via a direct dose-dependent toxicity. TMA can develop during the first few weeks of treatment and usually resolves with discontinuation of the drug.[10] In many reports, ciclosporin- and tacrolimus-induced TMA occurred in patients who may have had an underlying diagnosis of aHUS with recurrence post-transplant, raising the question of whether this was a drug toxicity or a recurrence of an acute TMA, as can be seen post-transplant in aHUS patients.

Secondary TMA

Many conditions other than TTP and HUS can present with TMA findings. The following may present with acute TMA findings and may need to be excluded clinically before a diagnosis of TTP or aHUS can be made.

Disseminated intravascular coagulation (DIC) occurs when procoagulant factors in the blood lead to the generation of intravascular thrombin which, in turn, leads to intravascular coagulation, multi-organ failure, bleeding and thrombocytopenia. DIC is characterized by thrombocytopenia associated with raised D-dimers. There is variable derangement of the coagulation profile, with prolonged prothrombin time (PT) and activated partial thromboplastin time (APTT) occurring in 50–60% cases.[11] Fibrinogen may be reduced in very severe DIC. The International Society of Thrombosis and Haemostasis DIC scoring system is more than 90% sensitive and specific, provides an objective measurement of DIC and is predictive of mortality.[12]

Systemic infections. Other than STEC, TMA can be seen secondary to severe *Streptococcus pneumoniae* infection with either severe pneumonia or meningitis; it is usually seen in children. The mechanism of injury is possibly via the production of a bacterial neuraminidase that removes sialic acid from cell-surface glycoproteins, exposing Thomsen–Friedenreich antigen (T-antigen), leaving it to bind naturally occurring antibodies that fix complement, causing hemolysis and renal injury.[13]

Solid organ and stem-cell transplant TMA. TMA may occur through a mixture of mechanisms, including drug toxicity from the immunosuppressing agents mentioned above, severe infections or, in the case of hematopoietic stem-cell transplantation, graft-versus-host disease. A TMA associated with stem-cell transplant that is clinically similar to aHUS also occurs.

Cancer. Secondary TMAs are usually seen in adenocarcinoma of the pancreas, lung, prostate, stomach, colon, ovary, breast or metastatic cancer of unknown primary site. These are usually associated with progressive or metastatic disease, commonly with hepatic involvement. Treatment should be directed, if possible, at the underlying malignancy.

Pregnancy-associated TMA. While pregnancy can trigger disease onset in patients with cTTP, iTTP and aHUS, pregnancy has its own TMA differential diagnosis, which includes pre-eclampsia, eclampsia, HELLP (hemolysis, elevated liver enzymes, low platelet count), acute fatty liver of pregnancy, abruptio placenta, amniotic fluid embolism and retained products of conception.[14]

Autoimmune disorders. TMA can occur in antiphospholipid syndrome (APS) and progressive systemic sclerosis, particularly in association with acute scleroderma, renal crisis and malignant hypertension.

Systemic lupus erythematosus can present similarly to iTTP in rare cases. Additionally, autoantibodies against ADAMTS13 are more likely to occur in individuals with a pre-existing diagnosis of SLE than in someone without an autoimmune disorder. ADAMTS13 activity in these cases would be low and patients are treated as other patients with iTTP, with additional intervention for the underlying SLE.[15] Moreover, common markers for SLE, such as antinuclear antibodies (ANA) and anti-double-strand (ds)DNA antibodies can be positive in TTP, causing confusion.

Cobalamin metabolic defects. A rare autosomal recessive condition caused by mutation in *MMACHC*, the gene encoding methylmalonic aciduria and homocystinuria type C protein, results in developmental delay, neurological symptoms, pulmonary hypertension, renal failure and TMA. The diagnosis typically becomes apparent in infancy, but the condition can also occur later in older children and, rarely, in adults.

Laboratory studies show elevated plasma methylmalonic acid and homocysteine levels with low plasma methionine and sufficient vitamin B12 levels. Patients respond to high doses of hydroxycobalamin and betaine to treat and prevent signs and symptoms of an acute TMA.[16]

Malignant hypertension. Many clinical features of TTP and HUS can be present in malignant hypertension, including MAHA, thrombocytopenia, renal insufficiency and neurological deficits.[17] To complicate matters further, aHUS can have accelerated hypertension as a clinical presentation.

Systemic causes of anemia and/or thrombocytopenia that mimic TMA

Myelodysplastic syndromes that can mimic TMA include clonal disorders with ineffective hematopoiesis and dysplastic bone marrow with peripheral blood cytopenias. Individuals are usually older, with risk factors such as chemotherapy, chemical or radiation exposure.

Megaloblastic anemia (vitamin B12 deficiency). The morphology of red cells and platelets plus severe hemolysis in severe vitamin B12 deficiency may mimic that of TMA. Laboratory findings include anemia, reticulocytosis and thrombocytopenia. Patients will respond promptly to B12 injections and further investigations to exclude pernicious anemia should be undertaken. Therefore, routine screening for B12 and folate levels should be undertaken in acute TMA presentations.

Sickle cell disease. A single point mutation in the β-globin gene results in abnormal hemoglobin, which leads to chronic hemolytic anemia, painful vaso-occlusive disease and damage in almost every organ. Anemia, thrombocytopenia and distorted red cells can be confused for a TMA process, though patients are usually diagnosed with sickle cell disease at an early age.

Hemophagocytic lymphohistiocytosis (HLH) is a life-threatening syndrome marked by excessive inflammation and tissue destruction. The hyperinflammatory immune state occurs because the normal downregulation of the immune system by activated macrophages and lymphocytes is absent.[18] HLH presents as a febrile illness associated with multiple organ involvement, splenomegaly, anemia, thrombocytopenia, liver function abnormalities, coagulopathy and neurological abnormalities, which can mimic TTP.

Heparin-induced thrombocytopenia (HIT) is immune mediated, occurs 5–10 days after exposure and is due to antibodies to platelet factor 4. HIT causes thrombocytopenia and platelet activation, leading to venous and arterial thrombi. It is a clinical diagnosis that can be screened for using the 4 T scoring system (thrombocytopenia > 50%, platelet count decrease 5–10 days after heparin exposure, thrombosis and lack of other causes for thrombocytopenia) and confirmed by testing for heparin-associated antibodies.

Paroxysmal nocturnal hemoglobinuria (PNH) is caused by mutation of *PIGA*, which encodes phosphatidylinositol glycan anchor biosynthesis class A. The mutation leads to the absence of CD55 and CD59 from the surface of red cells, making them vulnerable to destruction by the complement system. Patients present with episodic hemolysis, bone marrow aplasia and thrombosis, and have an increased risk of leukemia or myelodysplasia.

Differential diagnostic approach

Immune-mediated TTP. Once TMA is suspected, it is important to quickly rule out secondary TMA and other systemic causes of anemia and thrombocytopenia that mimic TMA. Hematology consultation should be obtained early. Given the high mortality associated with untreated TTP, the challenging nature of the diagnosis and the typical several-days turnaround time for ADAMTS13 activity test results, the approach to a patient with suspected TTP often involves empiric treatment with plasma exchange and corticosteroids prior to confirmation of the diagnosis from ADAMTS13 activity. Assessing the response to plasma exchange (iTTP typically responds to plasma exchange therapy while aHUS typically does not) in terms of a rising platelet count and declining lactate dehydrogenase, in addition to the ADAMTS13 activity, can confirm the diagnosis.[6]

The finding of ADAMTS13 activity below 10 IU/dL confirms the diagnosis of TTP. Normal ADAMTS13 activity should lead to the consideration of other forms of TMA as a diagnosis, while intermediately low ADAMTS13 activity (between 10 and 20 IU/dL) needs to be interpreted carefully and may still be consistent with a diagnosis of TTP.

Congenital TTP is much less common than iTTP. The prevalence is approximately 1 per million and cTTP accounts for a small percentage of TTP diagnoses. The suspicion for cTTP will also depend on age at presentation. The diagnosis of cTTP is made with the finding of undetectable ADAMTS13 activity (< 10 IU/dL) but with no clearly detectable inhibitor or anti-ADAMTS13 antibody. Mutation studies can then be used to confirm a cTTP diagnosis. In women of childbearing years, approximately 34% of newly diagnosed TTP cases during pregnancy will be cTTP, with pregnancy serving as the trigger for the acute TMA in individuals with previously undiagnosed congenital ADAMTS13 deficiency.[19]

During early childhood, the differential diagnosis includes STEC-HUS, aHUS and secondary TMA associated with diseases of early childhood. All young children should be tested for STEC because a significant number of children with STEC-HUS may not have the classic presentation with diarrhea. Other diseases associated with hemolysis and/or thrombocytopenia should be included in the differential for cTTP in young children, including immune thrombocytopenia (ITP) and hemolytic disease of the fetus and newborn.

Immune thrombocytopenia is characterized by immune-mediated platelet destruction and impaired production. Childhood ITP is usually acute, often occurring after a viral infection or vaccination, and usually resolves spontaneously within weeks to months. TMA is not a common feature and anemia is not pronounced unless there is significant bleeding. Neurological findings are not common unless there is intracranial hemorrhage, which can happen in severe thrombocytopenia.

Hemolytic disease of the fetus and newborn is caused by transplacentally transmitted maternal immunoglobulin (Ig)G directed against fetal red cell antigens, which causes hemolysis and the subduing of erythropoiesis. It presents with anemia, hyperbilirubinemia, extramedullary hematopoiesis and decreased haptoglobin, which can overlap with cTTP in severe cases. It is diagnosed by clinical history and is differentiated from TTP by lack of TMA findings.

Key points – differential diagnosis

- The thrombotic microangiopathies (TMAs) are a group of disorders that share common clinical characteristics and findings, but with differing pathobiologies that lead to the TMA presentation.
- Individuals with hemolytic uremic syndrome and atypical hemolytic uremic syndrome typically present with more severe renal injury or renal failure compared with individuals with thrombotic thrombocytopenic purpura.
- Quinine, ciclosporin and tacrolimus can induce TMAs via an immune-mediated mechanism (quinine) or dose-dependent toxicity.
- Systemic disorders that can secondarily present with TMA findings include disseminated intravascular coagulation, sepsis/infection and autoimmune disorders (systemic lupus erythematosus).
- Diseases that present with significant thrombocytopenia mimicking a systemic TMA that should be considered in the differential diagnosis include myelodysplasia, megaloblastic anemia, heparin-induced thrombocytopenia and paroxysmal nocturnal hemoglobinuria.

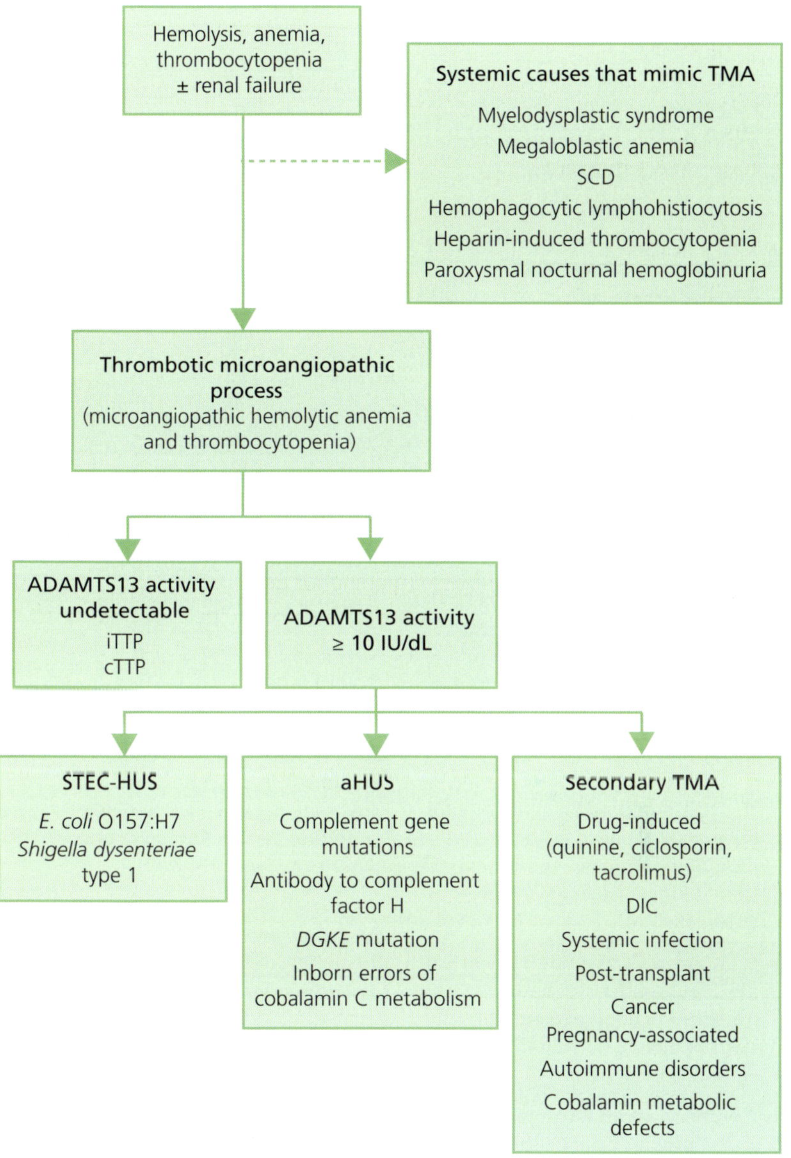

Figure 3.1 Differential diagnosis and pathway to evaluate the potential etiologies for thrombotic microangiopathic findings. aHUS, atypical hemolytic uremic syndrome; cTTP, congenital TTP; DIC, disseminated intravascular coagulation; iTTP, immune-mediated TTP; SCD, sickle cell disease; STEC-HUS, Shiga toxin-producing *Escherichia coli*-hemolytic uremic syndrome; TMA, thrombotic microangiopathy.

References

1. Tarr PI, Gordon CA, Chandler WL. Shiga-toxin-producing *Escherichia coli* and haemolytic uraemic syndrome. *Lancet* 2005;365:1073–86.

2. Tsai HM, Chandler WL, Sarode R et al. Von Willebrand factor and von Willebrand factor-cleaving metalloprotease activity in *Escherichia coli* O157:H7-associated hemolytic uremic syndrome. *Pediatr Res* 2001;49:653–9.

3. Wong CS, Mooney JC, Brandt JR et al. Risk factors for the hemolytic uremic syndrome in children infected with *Escherichia coli* O157:H7: A multivariable analysis. *Clin Infect Dis* 2012;55:33–41.

4. Loirat C, Fakhouri F, Ariceta G et al. An international consensus approach to the management of atypical hemolytic uremic syndrome in children. *Pediatr Nephrol* 2016; 31:15–39.

5. Taylor CM, Machin S, Wigmore SJ et al. Clinical practice guidelines for the management of atypical haemolytic uraemic syndrome in the United Kingdom. *Br J Haematol* 2010;148:37–47.

6. Cataland SR, Wu HM. How I treat: the clinical differentiation and initial treatment of adult patients with atypical hemolytic uremic syndrome. *Blood* 2014;123:2478–84.

7. Macia M, de Alvaro Moreno F, Dutt T et al. Current evidence on the discontinuation of eculizumab in patients with atypical haemolytic uraemic syndrome. *Clin Kidney J* 2017;10:310–19.

8. Al-Nouri ZL, Reese JA, Terrell DR et al. Drug-induced thrombotic microangiopathy: a systematic review of published reports. *Blood* 2015;125:616–18.

9. Dlott JS, Danielson CF, Blue-Hnidy DE, McCarthy LJ. Drug-induced thrombotic thrombocytopenic purpura/hemolytic uremic syndrome: a concise review. *Ther Apher Dial* 2004;8:102–11.

10. Remuzzi G, Bertani T. Renal vascular and thrombotic effects of cyclosporine. *Am J Kidney Dis* 1989;13:261–72.

11. Levi M, Toh CH, Thachil J, Watson HG. Guidelines for the diagnosis and management of disseminated intravascular coagulation. *Br J Haematol* 2009;145:24–33.

12. Wada H, Matsumoto T, Yamashita Y. Diagnosis and treatment of disseminated intravascular coagulation (DIC) according to four DIC guidelines. *J Intensive Care* 2014;2:15.

13. Copelovitch L, Kaplan BS. *Streptococcus pneumoniae*-associated hemolytic uremic syndrome. *Pediatr Nephrol* 2008;23:1951–6.

14. Lattuda A, Rossi E, Calzarossa C et al. Mild to moderate reduction of a von Willebrand factor cleaving protease (ADAMTS-13) in pregnant women with HELLP microangiopathic syndrome. *Haematologica* 2003;88:1029–34.

15. Güngör T, Furlan M, Lämmle B et al. Acquired deficiency of von Willebrand factor-cleaving protease in a patient suffering from acute systemic lupus erythematosus. *Rheumatology* 2001;40:940–2.

16. Carrillo-Carrasco N, Chandler RJ, Venditti CP. Combined methylmalonic acidemia and homocystinuria, cblC type I. Clinical presentations, diagnosis and management. *J Inherit Metab Dis* 2012;35:91–102.

17. Van den Born BJ, van der Hoeven NV, Groot E et al. Association between thrombotic microangiopathy and reduced ADAMTS13 activity in malignant hypertension. *Hypertension* 2008;51:862–6.

18. Filipovich A, McClain K, Grom A. Histiocytic disorders: recent insights into pathophysiology and practical guidelines. *Biol Blood Marrow Transplant* 2010;16(Suppl):S82–9.

19. Mariotte E, Azoulay E, Galicier L et al. Epidemiology and pathophysiology of adulthood-onset thrombotic microangiopathy with severe ADAMTS13 deficiency (thrombotic thrombocytopenic purpura): a cross-sectional analysis of the French national registry for thrombotic microangiopathy. *Lancet Haematol* 2016;3:e237–45.

4 Laboratory findings and diagnosis

Jin-sup Shin MD, University College London Hospitals NHS Foundation Trust, London, UK

Thrombotic thrombocytopenic purpura (TTP) is an acute life-threatening thrombotic microangiopathy (TMA) that requires rapid diagnosis and treatment. The TMAs are a group of disorders characterized by microangiopathic hemolytic anemia (MAHA), thrombocytopenia and occlusive micro- and macrovascular thrombosis.

A number of medical conditions present with TMA, including:

- fibrin-platelet thrombosis, most commonly seen in disseminated intravascular coagulation (DIC) but also occasionally seen in catastrophic antiphospholipid syndrome, heparin-induced thrombocytopenia (HIT) and HELLP (hemolysis, elevated liver enzymes and low platelet count) syndrome
- von Willebrand factor (VWF)-platelet thrombosis, seen with severe ADAMTS13 deficiency in TTP (immune-mediated and congenital subtypes) and characterized by the presence of ultra-large VWF multimers and VWF- and platelet-rich thrombi in arterioles and capillaries[1]
- endothelial inflammation/damage with fibrinoid necrosis, seen in hemolytic uremic syndrome (HUS); intraluminal thrombosis is frequently present
- inflammatory vasculopathy/vasculitis, in which changes can involve endothelial cells and intima, though it may be autoimmune (for example, systemic lupus erythematosus, scleroderma)
- intravascular clusters of cancer cells (tumor cell embolism), as occurs in advanced cancer.

Differentiating these conditions from TTP can be difficult because of the clinical overlap in presenting features; frequently, other more common TMAs need to be excluded (see chapter 3). This is particularly important as treatments for these disorders differ, and not all benefit from plasma exchange. Furthermore, early effective treatment in TTP is associated with improved clinical outcomes.[2] A summary of the approach to diagnosing TTP is shown in Figure 4.1 at the end of this chapter.

Diagnosing TTP

TTP was originally characterized by a pentad of thrombocytopenia, MAHA, fluctuating neurological signs, renal impairment and fever. However, advances in our understanding have demonstrated that TTP can present without the full pentad.

TTP is now defined by MAHA with moderate-to-severe thrombocytopenia and associated organ dysfunction (neurological, cardiac, gastrointestinal and renal involvement) without an alternative explanation. The diagnosis is confirmed by an ADAMTS13 activity level below 10 IU/dL. Table 4.1 lists the investigations that should be performed for an individual with a suspected diagnosis of TTP.

Typical laboratory findings. Platelet consumption by platelet-rich thrombi results in thrombocytopenia. The median platelet count is typically 10–30 × 10^9/L at presentation. Median hemoglobin levels on admission are 80–100 g/L, with evidence of MAHA (schistocytes in the blood film, low haptoglobin, raised reticulocyte counts and raised lactate dehydrogenase [LDH] levels).[3–5] The direct antiglobulin (Coombs) test is negative. Acute renal failure (requiring hemodialysis) is rare in immune-mediated TTP (iTTP), with a median creatinine level at presentation of 90 μmol/L (1.0 mg/dL). Significant renal impairment usually points to a diagnosis of HUS.[6] The coagulation screen (prothrombin time, activated partial thromboplastin time and fibrinogen) is usually normal as well.

Cardiac involvement is common in iTTP, with troponin being raised in 60% of cases. It is a sign of poor prognosis, being associated with a sevenfold increase in mortality rate compared with TTP patients with normal troponin levels.

Neurological impairment is also common, with symptoms ranging from headaches and altered personality to strokes, seizures and a fluctuating level of consciousness, including coma. A reduced Glasgow Coma Scale (GCS) score is a worrying feature as it is associated with an increase in mortality. CT or MRI of the brain should be considered in these patients, but it is important that imaging on admission should not interrupt plasma exchange therapy.

Precipitating cause. Investigations should also be tailored toward looking for a precipitating cause. If clinically indicated, blood, urine and stool cultures should be sent to exclude infection. A stool culture

TABLE 4.1

Investigations and expected results for patients with a suspected diagnosis of TTP*

Investigations for diagnosis	Expected findings in TTP
Full blood count and blood film	Anemia, thrombocytopenia, schistocytes
Reticulocyte count	Raised
Haptoglobin	Reduced
Coagulation screen (PT, aPTT, fibrinogen)	Normal
Renal profile	Renal impairment in ~ 20–30% of cases
Troponin T/I	Raised in ~ 60% of cases
Liver function tests	Raised bilirubin (hemolysis)
Lactate dehydrogenase	Raised
Direct antiglobulin test	Negative
Hepatitis A/B/C and HIV tests	Prior to plasma therapy and to exclude viral precipitant
ADAMTS13 activity and anti-ADAMTS13 IgG	ADAMTS13 activity < 10 IU/dL iTTP: raised anti-ADAMTS13 IgG cTTP: reduced/absent IgG
CT/MRI brain	To determine neurological involvement
Investigations for secondary causes	
Autoantibody screen (ANA, RF, LA, ACLA)	Exclude autoimmune disease
Urine/serum HCG	Exclude pregnancy (in all women of childbearing age)
Microbiology: blood, urine, stool culture	Screen for infection, including Shiga toxin (if diarrhea at presentation)
CT thorax/abdomen/pelvis ± tumor markers	Exclude underlying malignancy

*Samples should be sent for investigations prior to plasma exchange.
ACLA, anticardiolipin antibody; ANA, antinuclear antibody; aPTT, activated partial thromboplastin time; cTTP, congenital TTP; HCG, human chorionic gonadotropin; IgG, immunoglobulin G; iTTP, immune-mediated TTP; LA, lupus antibody; PT, prothrombin time; RF, rheumatoid factor.
Adapted from Scully et al. 2012.[3]

can rule out an important differential diagnosis, infection-associated HUS, which is typically associated with Shiga toxin-producing *Escherichia coli* (STEC) and may present with bloody diarrhea, TMA and marked renal impairment. Unlike TTP, management is usually supportive rather than with plasma exchange.

Other precipitating causes to be excluded are autoimmune disorders and pregnancy. A virology screen should be undertaken prior to exposure to plasma products, to exclude HIV and other viral-associated TTP.

Confirming the diagnosis

Once a diagnosis of TTP is suspected, treatment with plasma exchange should be initiated without delay. Prior to therapy, blood samples should be taken for ADAMTS13 assays, specifically:

- ADAMTS13 activity
- functional inhibitor based on mixing studies ± anti-ADAMTS13 immunoglobulin (Ig)G.

ADAMTS13 activity level below 10 IU/dL confirms the diagnosis of TTP. Samples taken immediately following plasma therapy may give a falsely elevated ADAMTS13 activity. However, it has been shown that in more than 78% of cases, samples taken after 3 days of plasma exchange still had an ADAMTS13 activity level below 10 IU/dL.[7] The presence of an inhibitor on mixing studies or anti-ADAMTS13 IgG may help to confirm the diagnosis of iTTP in these situations. Other TMAs, by definition, will not have an ADAMTS13 activity below 10 IU/dL or the presence of significant anti-ADAMTS13 IgG.

Congenital TTP (Upshaw–Schulman syndrome). A persistent deficiency (< 10 IU/dL) of ADAMTS13 activity, with no evidence of inhibitory autoantibodies, suggests a diagnosis of cTTP. Individuals can present in the neonatal period, childhood or adulthood, with presentation typically associated with a trigger, such as infection, vaccination or pregnancy.[8] The diagnosis is confirmed by molecular demonstration of a pathogenic homozygous or compound heterozygous mutation in the *ADAMTS13* gene (see chapter 1). Family members undergoing genetic testing should receive genetic counseling, as many mutations are of unknown significance – even if gene variants are detected, family members may be normal with no symptoms of TTP.

Immune-mediated TTP can be categorized according to the presence (secondary iTTP) or absence (primary iTTP) of a precipitating factor. Both groups are defined by ADAMTS13 activity below 10 IU/dL and the presence of ADAMTS13 autoantibodies. Both also require immediate therapy with plasma exchange and steroids.

Primary iTTP accounts for approximately two-thirds of iTTP cases. The remainder are secondary TTPs, of which the commonest causes are autoimmune disorders, infection, pregnancy, HIV and drugs (Table 4.2). Treatment of secondary iTTP can be tailored toward the underlying precipitant: for example, discontinuation of the implicated drug or highly active antiretroviral therapies (HAART) in HIV-associated TTP.

Screening for severe ADAMTS13 deficiency

A number of scoring systems have been developed to help predict the likelihood of severe deficiency of ADAMTS13 activity and differentiate TTP from other TMAs.[9–11] One example is the PLASMIC score (Table 4.3),

TABLE 4.2

Precipitating causes in immune-mediated TTP episodes

Precipitant	Frequency of TTP cases (%)
Idiopathic	59
Autoimmune disease	14
Infection	11
Pregnancy	7
Cancer	4
HIV	2
Drugs	1
Other	2

Source: TMA Registry of the French Reference Center.[5]

which is composed of seven elements: platelets, lysis, active cancer, stem-cell or organ transplant, mean cell volume (MCV), international normalized ratio (INR) and creatinine. In conjunction with clinical assessment, it calculates the risk of severe ADAMTS13 deficiency and therefore allows early rapid screening of patients who can benefit from plasma-based therapy.

The total score ranges from 0 to 7 points:

- 0–4: low risk of severe ADAMTS13 deficiency
- 5: intermediate risk of severe ADAMTS13 deficiency
- 6–7: high risk of severe ADAMTS13 deficiency.

Another predictive scoring system, developed by the French TMA Reference Center, consists of only three criteria: platelet count less than or equal to 30 × 10^9/L, serum creatinine less than or equal to 200 μmol/L (2.25 mg/dL) and presence of antinuclear antibodies (ANA).

TABLE 4.3

PLASMIC scoring system for predicting thrombotic microangiopathy associated with severe ADAMTS13 deficiency

Investigation	Points
Platelet count < 30 × 10^9/L	1
Hemolysis variable*	1
No active cancer	1
No history of solid-organ or stem-cell transplant	1
MCV < 90 × 10^{-15} L	1
INR < 1.5	1
Creatinine < 176 μmol/L†	1

*Reticulocyte count > 2.5% or undetectable haptoglobin or indirect bilirubin > 34.2 μmol/L (2.0 mg/dL). †2.0 mg/dL. INR, international normalized ratio; MCV, mean cell volume.
Source: Bendapudi et al. 2017.[11]

Internal validation of the scoring system demonstrated that when all three criteria were present, specificity was 98.1% and positive predictive value was 98.7%, minimizing the number of false-positive diagnoses. When at least one criterion was present, sensitivity was 98.8% (and negative predictive value was 93.3% [95% confidence interval 85.2–100%]), minimizing the number of false-negative diagnoses.

Although a creatinine level above 150–200 μmol/L (1.70–2.25 mg/dL) and a platelet count above 30 × 10^9/L usually exclude a diagnosis of severe ADAMTS13 deficiency,[10,12] there are a minority of people with TTP who present with platelet counts above 30 × 10^9/L or marked renal impairment. Basing therapy decisions on these cut-offs alone runs the risk of potentially missing these atypical presentations. Therefore, the diagnosis of TTP should be definitively confirmed by analysis of ADAMTS13 activity.

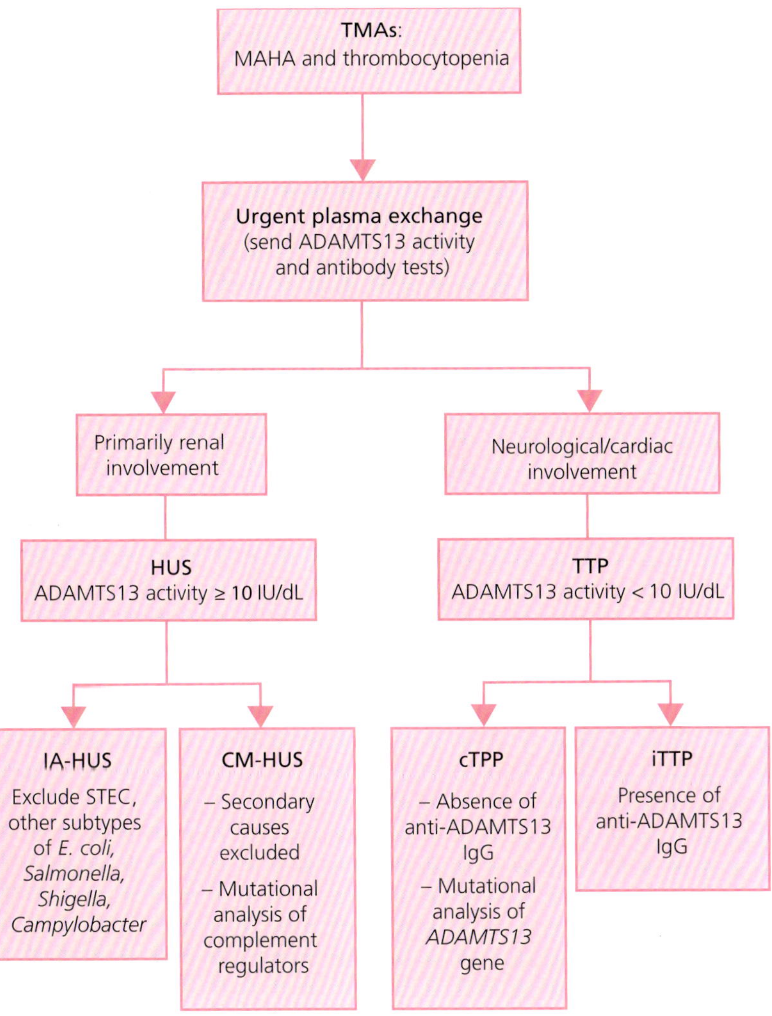

Figure 4.1 A summary of the approach to diagnosis of thrombotic thrombocytopenic purpura (TTP). Adapted from Scully 2017.[13] CM, complement-mediated; cTTP, congenital TTP; HUS, hemolytic uremic syndrome; IA, infection-associated; IgG, immunoglobulin G; iTTP, immune-mediated TTP; MAHA, microangiopathic hemolytic anemia; STEC, Shiga toxin-producing *Escherichia coli*; TMA, thrombotic microangiopathy.

Key points – laboratory findings and diagnosis

- Untreated thrombotic thrombocytopenic purpura (TTP) is associated with a high mortality rate; TTP should be treated as a medical emergency.
- Plasma exchange should be started without delay in an individual presenting with microangiopathic hemolytic anemia and thrombocytopenia in the absence of any other identifiable cause.
- Immune-mediated TTP is often associated with organ involvement, typically neurological and cardiac. Both are markers of poor prognosis and may identify higher-risk patients.
- Precipitating factors, such as HIV, autoimmune disease, drugs and pregnancy, should be excluded. Treatment should be tailored toward the underlying cause.
- Pretreatment samples should be sent for ADAMTS13 activity and anti-ADAMTS13 immunoglobulin (Ig)G levels. Plasma exchange should be started immediately afterward.
- Diagnosis of TTP is defined by an ADAMTS13 activity level below 10 IU/dL. A level of 10 IU/dL or higher is in keeping with atypical (complement-mediated) hemolytic uremic syndrome and other thrombotic microangiopathies.
- Immune-mediated TTP is confirmed with elevated anti-ADAMTS13 IgG, whereas these antibodies are absent in congenital TTP.
- Scoring systems such as PLASMIC can be a useful tool for predicting the likelihood of severe deficiency of ADAMTS13 activity, especially in settings where ADAMTS13 assays are not readily available. However, wherever possible, definitive confirmation of TTP should be based on analysis of ADAMTS13 activity.

References

1. Tsai HM, Lian ECY. Antibodies to von Willebrand factor-cleaving protease in acute thrombotic thrombocytopenic purpura. *N Engl J Med* 1998;339:1585–94.

2. Scully M, Goodship T. How I treat thrombotic thrombocytopenic purpura and atypical haemolytic uraemic syndrome. *Br J Haematol* 2014;164:759–66.

3. Scully M, Hunt BJ, Benjamin S et al. Guidelines on the diagnosis and management of thrombotic thrombocytopenic purpura and other thrombotic microangiopathies. *Br J Haematol* 2012;158:323–35.

4. Scully M, Yarranton H, Liesner R et al. Regional UK TTP Registry: correlation with laboratory ADAMTS 13 analysis and clinical features. *Br J Haematol* 2008:142:819–26.

5. Mariotte E, Azoulay E, Galicier L et al. Epidemiology and pathophysiology of adulthood-onset thrombotic microangiopathy with severe ADAMTS13 deficiency (thrombotic thrombocytopenic purpura): a cross-sectional analysis of the French national registry for thrombotic microangiopathy. *Lancet Haematol* 2016;3:e237–45.

6. Hassan S, Westwood J, Ellis D et al. The utility of ADAMTS13 in differentiating TTP from other acute thrombotic microangiopathies: results from the UK TTP Registry. *Br J Haematol* 2015;171:830–5.

7. Wu N, Liu J, Yang S et al. Diagnostic and prognostic values of ADAMTS13 activity measured during daily plasma exchange therapy in patients with acquired thrombotic thrombocytopenic purpura. *Transfusion* 2015;55:18–24.

8. Scully M, Cataland S, Coppo P et al. Consensus on the standardization of terminology in thrombotic thrombocytopenic purpura and related thrombotic microangiopathies. *J Thromb Haemost* 2017;15:312–22.

9. Bentley MJ, Lehman CM, Blaylock RC et al. The utility of patient characteristics in predicting severe ADAMTS13 deficiency and response to plasma exchange. *Transfusion* 2010;50:1654–64.

10. Coppo P, Schwarzinger M, Buffet M et al. Predictive features of severe acquired ADAMTS13 deficiency in idiopathic thrombotic microangiopathies: the French TMA reference center experience. *PLoS One* 2010;5:e10208.

11. Bendapudi PK, Hurwitz S, Fry A et al. Derivation and external validation of the PLASMIC score for rapid assessment of adults with thrombotic microangiopathies: a cohort study. *Lancet Haematol* 2017;4:e157–64.

12. Zuber J, Fakhouri F, Roumenina LT et al. Use of eculizumab for atypical haemolytic uraemic syndrome and C3 glomerulopathies. *Nat Rev Nephrol* 2012;8:643–57.

13. Scully M. Thrombocytopenia in hospitalized patients: approach to the patient with thrombotic microangiopathy. *Hematology Am Soc Hematol Educ Program* 2017;2017:651–9.

5 Management

Salma Shaikhouni MD, Department of Medicine, Ohio State University, Columbus, OH, USA, and

Filadelfiya Zvinovski MD, Department of Medicine, Mt Carmel Health System, Columbus, OH, USA

Immune-mediated TTP

Once a diagnosis of thrombotic thrombocytopenic purpura (TTP) is strongly suspected, treatment must be initiated as soon as possible. Delays in initiating treatment have been associated with early mortality. Therefore, the initial management for a patient with suspected TTP will typically involve empiric plasma exchange therapy, which should usually be started before the diagnosis is confirmed.

Plasma exchange therapy. The introduction of plasma exchange therapy revolutionized the treatment of TTP. It remains the mainstay of acute TTP treatment. Nearly 90% of patients will survive an acute TTP episode with plasma exchange therapy whereas, in contrast, there was near uniform mortality prior to the discovery of its effectiveness in TTP. Because of this, it is imperative to start plasma exchange as soon as possible.

It is hypothesized that plasma exchange works via repletion of the ADAMTS13 protease and/or the removal of the pathologic autoantibodies that inhibit ADAMTS13 function. The volume of exchange and replacement fluid used for the exchange can vary by institution, and it is not clear if there are material differences between replacement products. In general, in the acute phase, plasma exchange should be performed daily, with 1 to 1.5 plasma volume exchanges for the first few days; some centers use higher volume exchanges (1.5 plasma volume) for the initial days before dropping to one plasma volume exchanges thereafter for patients with a more severe presentation. For refractory or resistant cases, twice-daily exchanges can be considered, but this approach is less well supported by evidence.[1]

Plasma exchange should be continued until disease response is achieved; response is defined as a platelet count above 150×10^9/L for two consecutive days. The expected response to plasma exchange would be a gradual decline in lactate dehydrogenase (LDH) followed by an increase in platelet count. This provides reassurance that the patient is responding well to therapy. A clinical response (platelet count > 150 × 10^9/L) would be expected 4–6 days after starting plasma exchange therapy.[2]

In the absence of convincing data, the most effective method of stopping plasma exchange has been debated. There have been advocates of tapering to reduce the rates of early recurrence/exacerbation and relapse, but no benefit has been established compared with stopping plasma exchange.[3] New approaches to therapy, including the use of caplacizumab (discussed below), that are able to prevent TTP exacerbations may make this issue less relevant in the future.

Glucocorticoids. It is hypothesized that glucocorticoids suppress antibody inhibitors of ADAMTS13 and thus may be an effective adjunct to plasma exchange. An early study in which steroids were given to treat TTP suggested efficacy, but the study was done before it became feasible to measure ADAMTS13 activity.[4] Glucocorticoids are now typically used in combination with plasma exchange as soon as a diagnosis of immune-mediated TTP (iTTP) is presumed.[1] There are, however, no randomized controlled trials that compare the efficacy of plasma exchange plus steroids with plasma exchange alone. A prospective randomized study comparing prednisone with ciclosporin as adjunct to plasma exchange found no significant difference in exacerbation rates between the two arms, but did show a decrease in anti-ADAMTS13 antibodies and improvement in ADAMTS13 activity in the first month after stopping plasma exchange that was significantly better in the prednisone arm compared with the ciclosporin arm.[5]

Intravenous methylprednisolone,1 g/day, has been recommended in severe disease.[6] High-dose oral prednisolone at 1 mg/kg/day can be considered in less severe disease without neurological or cardiac involvement. Steroid treatments are typically continued throughout plasma exchange therapy. Once plasma exchange is completed and clinical response is achieved, steroids should be tapered and discontinued over 3–4 weeks.

Rituximab has been used increasingly in recent years as more data have accumulated to demonstrate its efficacy in patients with refractory or relapsing TTP. Rituximab is most commonly given intravenously at a dose of 375 mg/m^2 weekly for 4 weeks. It is typically given immediately after plasma exchange to minimize its clearance by the procedure. The efficacy of rituximab is based on its ability to clear the B cells that produce anti-ADAMTS13 immunoglobulin (Ig)G. At least 1–2 weeks are required for the rituximab to exert its effect and improve ADAMTS13 activity.[7] The best available data suggest that it should be used in patients with refractory or poorly responding disease, as well as those with a prior history of relapses and a relapsing TTP phenotype. However, phase II trials of rituximab as a first-line treatment for TTP, in conjunction with plasma exchange and steroid, suggest that earlier upfront rituximab leads to shorter hospitalizations.[7]

Caplacizumab is a nanobody (antibody fragment that has the structural and functional properties of naturally occurring heavy-chain-only antibodies) that targets the A1 domain of von Willebrand factor (VWF). By binding to VWF, caplacizumab blocks the ability of VWF to bind platelets, inhibiting the formation of microthrombi in TTP. It has no effect on the formation of autoantibodies to ADAMTS13. Caplacizumab was approved by both European Union and US regulatory authorities for the treatment of TTP in conjunction with plasma exchange and immune suppression. Trials have demonstrated a faster platelet response, but, more importantly, caplacizumab has been shown to significantly decrease the exacerbation rate (recurrence of TTP in the first month after stopping plasma exchange) after the acute TTP episode. This provides effective protection from recurrence for the patient until immunosuppressive therapy can improve the patient's ADAMTS13 activity.

The primary side effect associated with the use of caplacizumab is an increase in the risk of bleeding, especially mucocutaneous bleeding. The bleeding symptoms that were reported in the clinical trials were typically mild and manageable. VWF concentrates can be used as an antidote to treat any bleeding symptoms that develop.[8]

Supportive care during acute episodes. During the acute phase, complete blood count (CBC) and LDH should be monitored daily to help judge the response to immunosuppressive and plasma exchange therapy. Packed red blood cell transfusions should be administered as needed to keep the hemoglobin over 70 g/L (7.0 g/dL) during plasma exchange; folic acid supplementation is also indicated because of the high cell turnover in active hemolysis. Platelet transfusions should not be routinely used in patients with TTP; they should only be considered in cases of significant clinical bleeding. Pharmacological prophylaxis for deep vein thrombosis is also indicated when it is safe to administer, typically when the platelet count has increased above 50×10^9/L. Low-dose aspirin daily should also be administered when it is safe to do so in cases of cardiac involvement, as assessed by symptoms or elevated cardiac enzymes.

Disease-response definitions. A consensus panel of TTP experts was convened to draw up clinical-response definitions that can be used in both clinical research and the clinical care of patients (Table 5.1).[9]

TABLE 5.1
Clinical-response definitions

Clinical response: an increase in platelet levels above 150×10^9/L and an LDH that is less than ×1.5 ULN

Clinical remission: achieved when the criteria for clinical response are achieved and maintained for at least 30 days after the last plasma exchange

Exacerbation: a recurrent thrombocytopenia in the first 30 days after the last plasma exchange

Relapse: a new distinct TTP episode that occurs more than 30 days after the last plasma exchange

LDH, lactate dehydrogenase; ULN, upper limit of normal.
Source: Scully et al. 2017.[9]

Refractory TTP has been defined as a persistent thrombocytopenia, the lack of a sustained platelet count increment or a platelet count $< 50 \times 10^9$/L and an elevated LDH despite five plasma exchanges and steroid treatment. Treatment for refractory TTP should be tailored, based on response to initial therapy, but consideration should be given to:

- increasing the frequency of plasma exchange to twice daily
- switching to larger plasma volumes
- changing the steroid to intravenous methylprednisolone, 1 g/day.

Administer rituximab if not used already, keeping in mind that it may take at least 1–2 weeks for a meaningful response to occur.[7,10,11] Additional treatments that have been reported to have efficacy for refractory TTP include both ciclosporin and bortezomib.[11,12]

Congenital TTP

Acute treatment. The mainstay is plasma infusion to replace the deficient ADAMTS13 protease. Patients with cTTP do not have an ADAMTS13 autoantibody that needs to be removed, and therefore plasma exchange is not required. Some individuals with cTTP may require only intermittent plasma infusions to treat acute episodes, while others may require ongoing prophylactic therapy to prevent symptoms and treat ongoing microangiopathic findings.

A typical initial plasma dose is 10–15 mL/kg, which should provide an ADAMTS13 activity level of 25–37 IU/dL, assuming a plasma volume of 40 mL/kg. Patients are infused daily until the platelet count recovers to normal, which may require only 1–3 days of plasma infusion.[13] Patients with cTTP may have complete resolution of symptoms after plasma infusion. The half-life of ADAMTS13 in the circulation is approximately 2.5 days. We use a normal platelet count (typically $> 150 \times 10^9$/L) as a marker of resolution of acute thrombotic microangiopathy (TMA) and microvascular thrombi.[1]

Another treatment option is factor VIII concentrate products that contain variable amounts of ADAMTS13. Virally inactivated intermediate purity factor VIII concentrates, such as type 8Y, have been used to treat cTTP in several studies. Successful dosing regimens include 15–30 U/kg of 8Y, but the lack of consistent ADAMTS13 concentrations means that the ADAMTS13 dose administered is uncertain. Antibodies to ADAMTS13 have not been detected following the use of 8Y.[14] Another plasma-derived factor VIII concentrate, Koate, has also been used successfully in cTTP.

Chronic treatment. Patients with cTTP with ongoing TTP activity may need to be maintained on prophylactic plasma infusions to prevent persistent TMA findings and treat symptoms. Prophylactic plasma infusions may be administered at a dose of 10–15 mL/kg every 2–3 weeks,[13] with changes in dosage based on symptoms and/or platelet counts and ability to handle the infusion volume. Individuals who experience symptoms with this schedule may benefit from increasing the dose and/or shortening the interval between doses.[15]

Some cTTP patients experience repeated episodes of thrombocytopenia, microangiopathic hemolytic anemia and end-organ injury, including neurological symptoms (headaches, syncopal episodes, lethargy), renal insufficiency and abdominal pain.[15] Prophylactic therapy with plasma infusions is often a lifetime commitment. This therapy is appropriate to continue if patients benefit from improved symptoms after plasma infusion. Patients may notice improvements in their quality of life, with more energy and decreased frequency of headaches.

Prophylactic therapy requires the patient to have intravenous access and increases patient burden in travel time and costs, as well as potential transfusion reactions. Therefore, offering patients the alternative of close monitoring for symptoms without treatment is sometimes appropriate. Moreover, patients who were diagnosed by genetic testing of family members but who have never had an acute episode may need only close monitoring and not prophylactic plasma infusions. It is also appropriate to avoid prophylactic plasma infusions in patients who have had a clear trigger for their TTP episode (physiological stress or infection) that has been addressed and is no longer present. These patients may avoid the time commitment and potential complications associated with long-term plasma infusion therapy.

Routine monitoring. Individuals with cTTP require lifelong monitoring for symptoms of microvascular thrombosis, including headaches, syncopal episodes and other neurological symptoms.

Even if the platelet count is above 150 × 10^9/L, individuals may still have symptoms attributed to TTP that resolve with treatment with plasma infusions.

Patients should be immediately started on plasma infusion therapy if they experience unexplained neurological findings or thrombocytopenia. For patients not on chronic plasma therapy, routine CBC is not required unless the patient has symptoms that could be attributable to TTP (headaches, other unexplained neurological symptoms, abdominal pain, lethargy) or a generalized illness (e.g. upper respiratory tract infection, urinary tract infection). In these cases, a CBC and other measures of hemolysis (peripheral smear review, increased LDH) might confirm the need for plasma therapy.

Monitoring during pregnancy. Planning for pregnancy should be a routine component of care for women of childbearing potential, but it is especially important for women with cTTP who plan to become pregnant. Women with cTTP should be evaluated by a hematologist and maternal–fetal medicine specialist before becoming pregnant as pregnancy can trigger an episode. With appropriate guidance and therapy, women can have healthy and successful pregnancies.[16] It is recommended that women start prophylactic plasma infusions as soon as the pregnancy is confirmed. Plasma infusions of 10 mL/kg are administered every 2 weeks but may be increased to 15 mL/kg based on changes in the platelet count or symptoms. These treatments should continue biweekly for 6 weeks postpartum.[17]

Recombinant ADAMTS13 therapy. Although plasma infusions have proven to be an effective method of treating cTTP, there are still concerns about efficacy and the potential for long-term vascular and neurological events, even with prophylactic plasma infusions. A recent study of recombinant ADAMTS13 (rADAMTS13) has shown great promise. The rADAMTS13 was well-tolerated without serious adverse events or the development of neutralizing anti-rADAMTS13 antibodies from the initial single-dose study.[18] In this study, the in vivo function of rADAMTS13 was demonstrated by the cleavage of ultra-large VWF multimers and an increase in the platelet count. The rADAMTS13 pharmacokinetics were comparable to those seen in plasma infusion studies, with evidence of pharmacodynamic activity.

Key points – management

- In patients presenting with a clinical picture consistent with an acute episode of thrombotic thrombocytopenic purpura (TTP), plasma exchange should be started empirically before the diagnosis is confirmed by ADAMTS13 activity testing.
- Glucocorticoid therapy to suppress the production of anti-ADAMTS13 antibodies is an important adjunct to plasma exchange therapy.
- Rituximab has an increasing role in the treatment of refractory and chronic relapsing TTP and may prevent future episodes by correcting the deficiency of ADAMTS13 activity.
- The development of caplacizumab as an adjunct to plasma exchange therapy has been shown to decrease the number of plasma exchange procedures required to achieve a normal platelet count and significantly decrease the risk for exacerbations of TTP.
- Many patients with congenital TTP require chronic plasma infusions as well as careful observations for chronic neurological and vascular complications.

References

1. Scully M, Goodship T. How I treat thrombotic thrombocytopenic purpura and atypical haemolytic uraemic syndrome. *Br J Haematol* 2014;164:759–66.

2. Peyvandi F, Scully M, Kremer Hovinga JA et al. Caplacizumab for acquired thrombotic thrombocytopenic purpura. *N Engl J Med* 2016;374:511–22.

3. Bandarenko N, Brecher ME. United States Thrombotic Thrombocytopenic Purpura Apheresis Study Group (US TTP ASG): multicenter survey and retrospective analysis of current efficacy of therapeutic plasma exchange. *J Clin Apher* 1998;13:133–41.

4. Bell WR, Braine HG, Ness PM et al. Improved survival in thrombotic thrombocytopenic purpura-hemolytic uremic syndrome. Clinical experience in 108 patients. *N Engl J Med* 1991;325:398–403.

5. Cataland SR, Kourlas PJ, Yang S et al. Cyclosporine or steroids as an adjunct to plasma exchange in the treatment of immune-mediated thrombotic thrombocytopenic purpura. *Blood Adv* 2017;1:2075–82.

6. Scully M, Hunt BJ, Benjamin S et al. Guidelines on the diagnosis and management of thrombotic thrombocytopenic purpura and other thrombotic microangiopathies. *Br J Haematol* 2012;158:323–35.

7. Scully M, McDonald V, Cavenagh J et al. A phase 2 study of the safety and efficacy of rituximab with plasma exchange in acute acquired thrombotic thrombocytopenic purpura. *Blood* 2011;118:1746–53.

8. Scully M, Cataland SR, Peyvandi F et al. Caplacizumab treatment for acquired thrombotic thrombocytopenic purpura. *N Engl J Med* 2019;380:335–46.

9. Scully M, Cataland S, Coppo P et al. Consensus on the standardization of terminology in thrombotic thrombocytopenic purpura and related thrombotic microangiopathies. *J Thromb Haemost* 2017;15:312–22.

10. Scully M, Cohen H, Cavenagh J et al. Remission in acute refractory and relapsing thrombotic thrombocytopenic purpura following rituximab is associated with a reduction in IgG antibodies to ADAMTS-13. *Br J Haematol* 2007;136:451–61.

11. Enami T, Suzuki T, Ito S et al. Successful treatment of refractory thrombotic thrombocytopenic purpura with cyclosporine and corticosteroids in a patient with systemic lupus erythematosus and antibodies to ADAMTS13. *Intern Med* 2007;46:1033–7.

12. Shortt J, Oh DH, Opat SS. ADAMTS13 antibody depletion by bortezomib in thrombotic thrombocytopenic purpura. *N Engl J Med* 2013;368:90–2.

13. Barbot J, Costa E, Guerra M et al. Ten years of prophylactic treatment with fresh-frozen plasma in a child with chronic relapsing thrombotic thrombocytopenic purpura as a result of a congenital deficiency of von Willebrand factor-cleaving protease. *British J Haematol* 2001;113:649–51.

14. Scully M, Gattens M, Khair K et al. The use of intermediate purity factor VIII concentrate BPL 8Y as prophylaxis and treatment in congenital thrombotic thrombocytopenic purpura. *Br J Haematol* 2006;135:101–4.

15. Alwan F, Vendramin C, Liesner R et al. Characterization and treatment of congenital thrombotic thrombocytopenic purpura. *Blood* 2019;133:1644–51.

16. Jiang Y, McIntosh JJ, Reese JA et al. Pregnancy outcomes following recovery from acquired thrombotic thrombocytopenic purpura. *Blood* 2014;123:1674–80.

17. Epperla N, Hemauer K, Friedman et al. Congenital thrombotic thrombocytopenic purpura related to a novel mutation in ADAMTS13 gene and management during pregnancy. *Am J Hematol* 2016;91:644–6.

18. Scully M, Knobl P, Kentouche K et al. Recombinant ADAMTS-13: first-in-human pharmacokinetics and safety in congenital thrombotic thrombocytopenic purpura. *Blood* 2017;130:2055–63.

Useful resources

Registries

International

Hereditary TTP Registry
https://ttpregistry.net

Australia

Thrombotic Thrombocytopenia Purpura/Thrombotic Microangiopathies Registry (TTP/TMA)
www.monash.edu/medicine/sphpm/registries/ttp

UK

The United Kingdom Thrombotic Thrombocytopenic Purpura (TTP) Registry
www.uclh.nhs.uk/OurServices/ServiceA-Z/Cancer/CBD/TTP/TTPRegistry/Pages/Home.aspx

USA

Oklahoma TTP Registry (articles about)
https://ouhsc.edu/platelets/TTP/ttp publications.html

Patient support

Thrombotic Thrombocytopenic Purpura (TTP) Network
www.ttpnetwork.org.uk/

Oklahoma TTP-HUS Patient Support Group
https://ouhsc.edu/platelets/TTP/pt group meetings.html

Answering TTP
www.answeringttp.org

Index

acquired TTP *see* immune-mediated TTP
ADAMTS13 protein 7
 autoantibodies 8, 30, 41
 and diagnosis 26, 28, 33, 41, 42–3
 mutations 8–10, 19, 41
 in pregnancy 20
 recombinant 54
 replacement 52–3
adolescents 16–17
age 9, 16–17, 19
anemia
 MAHA 8, 12, 13, 18, 39, 51
 megaloblastic 31
antibiotics 27
aspirin 51
autoimmune diseases 17–18, 30
 see also immune-mediated TTP

blood tests 29, 39, 41, 43–4, 51, 54
bortezomib 52
brain damage 12, 13, 14–15, 19, 28, 39

cancer 30, 38
caplacizumab 50
cardiac damage 12, 13, 14–15, 39, 51
children 9, 16–17, 18
 differentials 27, 29, 30–1, 33–4
chronic disease 20, 53
ciclosporin 28–9, 52
clinical presentation 16–22, 39
cobalamin
 metabolic defects 30–1
 vitamin B12 deficiency 31
complement 26
congenital TTP (cTTP)
 diagnosis 33–4, 41
 epidemiology 7
 etiology 7, 8–10
 management 52–4
 presentation 18–21
corticosteroids 49, 52
creatinine 39, 43–4

diagnosis 38–46
 cTTP 33–4, 41
 delayed 19
 differentials 21, 25–35, 38
 iTTP 25, 32–3, 42
diarrhea-associated HUS 16, 25–7, 33, 41
disseminated intravascular coagulation 29
drug-induced TMA 28–9, 42

eculizumab 28
elderly patients 16, 19
end-organ damage
 in HUS 25–6, 27, 28
 in TTP 12, 14–16, 17, 19, 25, 39, 51
epidemiology 7–8, 9, 12, 16, 27
etiology 8–10, 16, 20

factor VIII concentrate 52–3
familial TTP *see* congenital TTP
females *see* women
fetal loss 21
fever 14–15

gastrointestinal damage 13, 14–15, 16
gender 8, 12
genetics (ADAMTS13 mutations) 8–10, 19, 41
glucocorticoids 49, 52

heart damage 12, 13, 14–15, 39, 51
hemolytic disease of the fetus and newborn 33–4
hemolytic uremic syndrome (HUS) 38
 atypical 27–8
 STEC 16, 25–7, 33, 41
hemophagocytic lymphohistiocytosis 31–2
heparin-induced thrombocytopenia 32
hereditary TTP *see* congenital TTP

imaging 39
immune thrombocytopenia 33
immune-mediated TTP (iTTP)
 diagnosis 25, 32–3, 42
 epidemiology 8
 etiology 8
 management 41, 42, 48–52
 presentation 16, 17
infections 27, 29, 39–41

kidney damage *see* renal damage

lactate dehydrogenase (LDH) 39, 49, 52
late-onset cTTP 16, 19, 20–1

malignant hypertension 31
management 48–55
aHUS 28
cTTP 52–4
iTTP 41, 42, 48–52
STEC-HUS 27
methylprednisolone 49, 52
microangiopathic hemolytic anemia (MAHA) 8, 12, 13, 18, 39, 51
monitoring 53–4
myelodysplastic syndromes 31

neurological damage 12, 13, 14–15, 19, 28, 39

paroxysmal nocturnal hemoglobinuria 32
pathogenesis 7, 8–10, 20
pediatrics *see* children
plasma exchange 28, 32, 41, 48–9, 52
plasma infusions 52, 53, 54
PLASMIC score 33
platelet count 32, 39, 43–4, 48–9, 52
platelet transfusions 51
pre-eclampsia 20
prednisolone 49
pregnancy 9, 20–1, 30, 33, 54
presentation 16–22, 39
pyrexia 14–15

quinine 28

red blood cell transfusions 51
refractory TTP 50, 52
relapsing TTP 50
renal damage
HUS 25–6, 27, 28
TTP 14–15, 16, 19, 39
rituximab 50, 52

sex 8, 12
Shiga toxin-producing *E. coli*-HUS (STEC-HUS) 16, 25–7, 33, 41
sickle cell disease 31
steroids 49, 52
Streptococcus pneumoniae 29
subacute cTTP 20
supportive care 51
symptoms and signs 12–22, 39
systemic lupus erythematosus (SLE) 17, 30
tacrolimus 28–9
thrombocytopenia 12, 13, 18, 32, 33, 39
thromboprophylaxis 51
thrombotic microangiopathy (TMA) 8, 18, 38
drug-induced 28–9
HUS 25–8, 33
mimics 31–2
secondary 26, 29–31
transplant-related TMA 29–30
treatment *see* management
triggers 16, 18, 20, 39–41, 42
troponin 12, 39

Upshaw–Schulman syndrome *see* congenital TTP

virology screens 41
vitamin B12 deficiency 31
von Willebrand factor (VWF) 8, 20, 38, 50

women 8, 12
pregnancy 9, 20–1, 30, 33, 54

Notes:

Notes:

Notes:

Notes: